# HUNGRY?

The innocent recipe book for
filling your family with good stuff

# HUNGRY?

## The innocent recipe book for filling your family with good stuff

FOURTH ESTATE • London

First published in Great Britain in 2011 by Fourth Estate

An imprint of HarperCollins*Publishers*
77–85 Fulham Palace Road
London W6 8JB

2 4 6 8 9 7 5 3 1

The innocent wee-ometer first appeared in *Stay Healthy, Be Lazy*, a book we wrote
years ago and which is now worth quite a bit on that online auction site.

Bronte's amazing carrot cake recipe © Bronte Aurell 2011
Crumbs coconut macaroons recipe and Hot apple and cinnamon drink © Lucy and Claire Macdonald 2011
Ceri's mum's chocolate bran flake cakes recipe © Mrs Tallett 2011

Drinks recipes on pages 320–334 previously published in
*innocent smoothie recipe book* and *innocent little book of drinks*.

A catalogue record for this book is available from the British Library.

ISBN 978-0-00-741680-6

Printed and bound by Butler Tanner and Dennis Ltd, Frome and London, on recycled paper.

Read in your kitchen by you.

NOTE: This is a cookery book with lots of stuff to do, make and eat.
It is only a work of fiction in parts and would be a sadder book without these bits.
Any resemblance to persons living or dead should be plainly apparent to them
and we'd like to thank them again for helping make this book what it is.

For our mums

# Credits

These people made this book:

**Recipes**
Anna Jones

**Text**
Ceri Tallett

**Photography**
Clare Shilland

**Food stylists**
Anna Jones
Emily Ezekiel

**Design**
Ben Williams
Julian Humphries
Rachel Smyth

**Watchful eye**
Tansy Drake
Dan Germain
Vanessa Hattersley
Richard Reed

**Commissioning editor**
Louise Haines

**Editors**
Georgia Mason
Elizabeth Woabank
Ione Walder

**Production**
Chris Gurney

# Contents

# Alternative contents

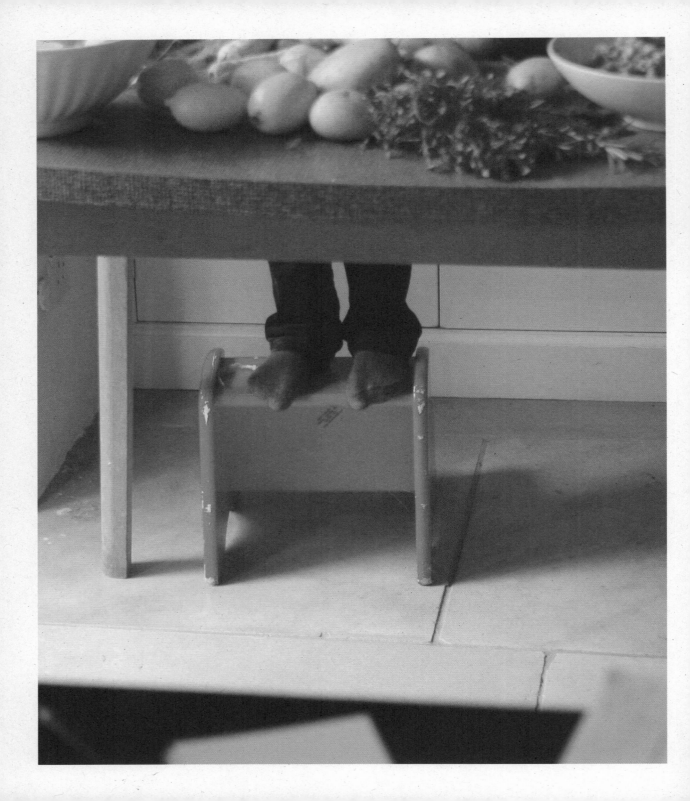

# Why have we written this book?

Hello. We're innocent and we make stuff that tastes good and does you good. We started by making smoothies in 1999 after the idea for the electric bath got binned. Since then we've moved into veg pots, healthy kids' drinks and the odd village fête.

We're now a bit older, wiser and (in some cases) beardier than when we started and some of us have even had babies. Which is sort of where the idea for this book came from.

Having sold our kids' smoothies in supermarkets across the land for the last 5 years, we had already bought into the benefits of getting fruit into small people. But when it came to finding a cook book to feed our families in a quick, tasty, nutritious way, there didn't seem to be any out there.

None that didn't involve spending hours labouring over the stove, making different meals for our kids or faffing about with miniature sushi.

So we decided to write our own.

Before we started, we asked the people who read our weekly newsletter what they thought. Hundreds of mums and dads got in touch to say they thought it was a very good idea and to suggest all sorts of recipes, tips and ideas on how to make it an all-round really useful tool.

So here it is: a guide to healthy, tasty, no-fuss food that the whole family can enjoy (and that doesn't take ages to make).

From classic family favourites and quick ideas for when you're in a hurry to posher stuff for when you're not, there's also loads of stuff for kids to do, make and help out with to get them involved and excited about food.

In other words, a book that makes it easy and tasty to get good stuff into your family. With no mini sashimi fiddling required whatsoever.

# How to use this book

There are several ways to use this book.

Each recipe has the steps where kids can get involved picked out in light grey to make it easy for them to help in the kitchen. These steps are just there as a guide, so if you're pushed for time, you can ignore them and get on with cooking by yourself.

In between the recipes, there are lots of distractions and ideas for your family to do while you're waiting for things to marinate, bake or just for the weather to cheer up.

At the front, there's an alternative contents page where we've divided recipes up into stuff like 'quick teas' for when you're in a hurry and 'leisurely cooking' for when you've got a bit more time on your hands (like breakfast at the weekends). So you can have a quick flick for ideas or plan in advance, depending on how busy you are.

There's a pocket at the back where you can keep together any recipes you pull out of magazines. Alternatively, feel free to use it as a 'safe place' to store important documents, petty cash or useful stuff like the washing machine instructions. That way, at least you'll always know where to go if the tumble dryer breaks. Plus burglars never look in the back of recipe books. Fact.

At the start of each recipe we've also highlighted how many fruit and veg portions there are per serving. Of all the recipes in this book, 85% contain at least one portion of fruit or veg, 10% contain fruit and veg that count towards your 5-a-day and the remaining 5% are treats to be respected as such. You can find out a bit more about fruit and veg portions on page 20.

# A quick guide to getting good stuff into small people

Our company purpose is to make natural, delicious food and drink that helps people live well and die old. It lies behind everything we make and this book is just as much a part of that mission as our smoothies, juice and veg pots.

We believe if you can get people on the right road from when they're knee-high and make it enjoyable along the way, it's more likely they'll stick on that path rather than deviating off down Takeaway Alley. Which is why getting kids involved in tasting, cooking and enjoying healthy, tasty food is the way forward. Chances are if they grew it, picked it, squashed it or stirred it, they're more likely to eat it.

But kids change their mind all the time. What they eat today, they might suddenly refuse to eat tomorrow. They don't obey the rules, they will nearly always want crisps over celery and, sometimes, you're just happy if they've eaten a spoonful of peas. It's not a personal slight – they're just experimenting with expressing opinions. So there's no point getting angry. It's like shouting at the bus driver when the bus is late – it won't change what time you get there. Far better to make the journey fun and interesting instead.

We know that health food has a reputation for being a bit of a boring, taste-free wilderness with only mung beans and flatulence for company. But that's not the stuff we're talking about. Healthy food done well is delicious.

So first and foremost, this book is about health through pleasure. To paraphrase Roald Dahl (a great advocate of little indulgences), treats are an essential part of life. We think you and your kids can eat well and still enjoy the odd slice of chocolate cake. Especially when it's got beetroot in it.

Ultimately, though, you're the best judge and example of what your kids should be eating. Of course, there will always be a perfect family next door who eat brown rice for breakfast, but your kids will base their habits on what you eat. So lead by example, get them cooking regularly and by the time they leave home, they'll hopefully be able to feed themselves properly and rustle you up a decent dinner while they are at it.

## Please say hello to Anna and Ness

Whilst we're very proud of all the stuff we make, in order to write a book like this, we thought it best to get some help from people who know a thing or two about writing recipes that actually work. So that's where Anna and Ness come in.

Anna Jones is a cook, writer and maker of beautiful looking (and tasting) food who has spent the last year working with us to help write the recipes for this book. Having trained at Fifteen, Anna then went off travelling round Spain, France and Italy, picking up cookery secrets on the way. Back in London, she's spent the last 7 years working for Jamie Oliver and is now busy doing lots of other interesting stuff with food as well as trying to surf (badly) and buying bits of old china for her kitchen.

Vanessa Hattersley is our nutritionist at Fruit Towers. She's in charge of giving the big official tick to all the stuff we make, ensuring that as well as tasting good, everything innocent makes does you good too. She's worked in the nutrition field for years (including for the NHS) and recently got top marks for her master's degree in food policy. Unlike the folk in those glossy telly ads, Ness doesn't wear a white coat, is a dab hand at baking and likes spending her evenings looking at stars through her telescope.

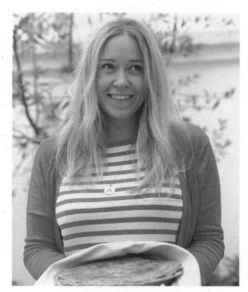

Anna and a pie

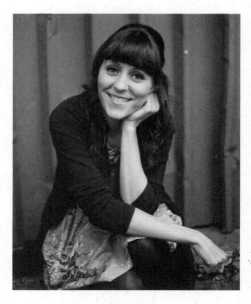

Ness and a fetching green door

# Do I need to buy any stuff?

Ingredients-wise, if you always try to have these things in your kitchen, along with an interesting mix of fruit and veg, then you should be ready for most recipes.

### Cupboard

Olive oil
Honey
Smoked paprika
Roasted peppers in a jar
Tinned tomatoes
Tinned pulses (chickpeas, kidney beans, lentils)

### Fridge

Eggs
Butter
Milk
Tomato purée
Mature Cheddar cheese
Parmesan cheese
Lemons
Plain yoghurt

### Freezer

Fresh herbs (snipped up)
Frozen mixed berries
Frozen veg (peas, spinach, sweetcorn)

## Equipment

If you only buy one thing for your kitchen, then let it be a food processor. It is the saver of time, the king of chopping and you can pretty much do anything in it – grate, julienne, purée, mix, salsa, pasa doble...

It'll save you money, time, washing up and having to buy a hundred other gadgets for your kitchen. The decent ones last for years so think of it as an investment/a helpful new member of your family.

Other good stuff to have on the Christmas list:

- **A pestle and mortar for bashing up spices** (or get yourself an electric coffee grinder).
- **Sharp knives**
  Sounds obvious but if they're blunt, they'll be rubbish.
- **An oil sprayer**
  Buying oil in an aerosol feels wrong and the stuff inside tastes like plastic. However, a quick spray of good olive oil is often all you need for cooking. So get yourself a smart oil sprayer, fill it with your favourite olive oil and let sloppy measuring and greasy dinners be a thing of the past.

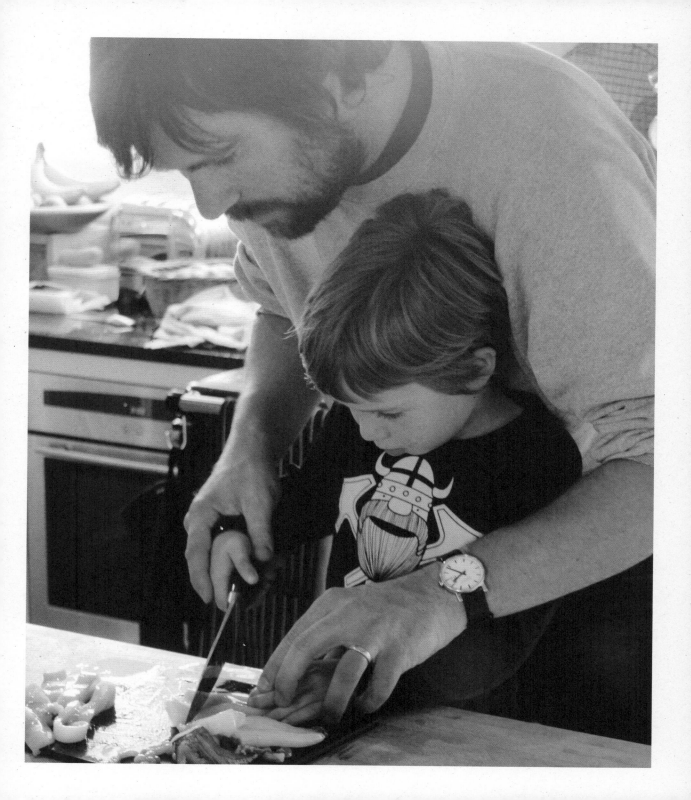

# A word or two on nutrition

We've kept this bit relatively simple, mainly because we're sure you already know most of the stuff there is to know about what to feed your kids.

Here are Ness's thoughts on getting good things into small people:

'Having worked as a nutritionist for many years now, I know how tricky it can be to get small people to eat healthy stuff, especially when there're so many brightly coloured, full-of-rubbish temptations out there.

'But good nutrition isn't difficult and eating healthily is pretty simple. Don't overdo it on the added fats and sugars. Eat lots of fruit and veg. Experiment with ingredients you might not have tried before. Remember to treat yourself and your kids. And try to cook from scratch wherever possible. That way you'll know what's gone into whatever you're eating.'

# A word on small tummies

A 5-year-old's stomach is somewhere around a quarter of the size of an adult's, yet they can need up to three-quarters of an adult's daily calories. So despite having smaller tummies, kids still need enough energy for all the running around they do as well as all the growth and development their bodies are doing. Thankfully, unlike grown-ups, kids are pretty good at judging how much food they need. So if you let them eat according to their appetite rather than forcing them to finish their plates, they shouldn't go wanting.

# A truly great plate

Aim for half your kid's plate to be filled with fruit and veg and the other half to be split between starchy foods (like brown bread, pasta, rice and spuds) and protein-based foods (like meat, fish, eggs and pulses).

The best way round the small tummies/fast growth rate thing is making sure your kids have regular meals and snacks throughout the day. This is especially important for pre-schoolers who grow much faster than kids over the age of 5. So for pre-schoolers, aim for 3 small meals and 2 to 3 snacks a day and for primary schoolers, aim for 3 meals and 1 or 2 snacks. By the time they get to secondary school, they're pretty much considered grown-ups in the nutrition world (minus the booze).

And don't forget drinking. Kids need to have 6 to 8 glasses of fluid every day. It doesn't have to be water, though try to keep any drinks with sugars (including fruit juice and smoothies) closer to mealtimes. Milk counts as fluid here too. Just in case you were wondering.

# So what's all this 5-a-day business?

The government tells us we need to eat at least 5 portions of a variety of fruit and veg every day as studies show that getting at least 400g a day can reduce the risk of developing heart disease and certain types of cancer.

The reason it's 5 portions as opposed to 3 or 7 is because an average serving size is said to be around 80g which divides neatly 5 times into 400g.

Since there are no official fruit and veg portion sizes for children, as a guide, go with one-third of an adult portion for pre-schoolers and half a portion for primary schoolers.

Here's a guide to what an adult portion of fruit or veg looks like:

- ½ a courgette, avocado or pepper
- 1 apple, banana, pear, orange, medium tomato, sweet potato, leek or corn-on-the-cob
- 150ml of juice
- 2 kiwi fruits, satsumas, plums, broccoli spears, carrots
- A big slice of pineapple, melon or papaya
- A tablespoon of dried fruit like raisins, sultanas and cranberries
- 3 tablespoons of any tinned fruit, pulses (chickpeas, lentils and kidney beans), peas, okra or sweetcorn (fresh, frozen or tinned)
- A big handful of grapes, fresh spinach, French beans or sugarsnap peas
- 7 strawberries, 4 dried apricots, 2 handfuls of mixed berries, 7 cherry tomatoes, 3 beetroots (cooked or fresh), a pudding bowl of salad leaves, 14 button mushrooms and 8 Brussels sprouts

The majority of the recipes in this book contain at least one portion per serving and there are lots of quick ideas for getting fruit and veg into your diet (without having to resort to cramming 3 carrots and a small leek down your neck before bed).

# Other bits and pieces

## Bread, rice, potatoes, spuds and starchy stuff

You want to have something from this group in every meal for kids, as this is where they're going to get most of their energy from. Breakfast is the best place to do this as after 10 hours' kip, the tank will be empty and kids will need lots of energy to get through the day and stay awake in double maths.

## Milk and dairy products

Dairy-wise, you should be aiming for around 3 servings per day from this group. Kids rely on milk for half of their calcium intake and the good news is that semi-skimmed milk has the same calcium content as whole milk. So if your child is eating well and growing properly, there's no problem moving them on to the semi-skimmed stuff after the age of 2. Wherever milk is mentioned in this book, though, we've left it up to you to decide what milk you use. As long as kids are drinking milk and not beer, we figure it's okay.

Cheese is slightly different. Despite us loving the stuff, when it comes to official portion sizes, we're not going to lie – a serving of cheese looks a bit measly when you measure it out. That's not nutritionists being mean. It's all to do with the high fat content of most cheeses. An adult's serving of cheese is 40g per day while kids should be eating around 25g. So be clever. Use mature Cheddar over mild (same amount of fat but bags more flavour). Top dishes with sprinklings and shavings rather than snowstorms. And never mix brie with tuna. Trust us.

## Meat, fish, eggs, pulses and all things protein

Very straightforward here. If your kids eat meat, go for 1 to 2 servings a day. Try to squeeze in fish a couple of times a week, especially the oily stuff as it's rich in omega-3 fats.

# All the stuff you worry about (also known as sugars and fats)

## Sugars

You can find sugars naturally in foods like fruit, veg and milk and you can also add sugar to food – like the sugar you put in your tea or the honey you squeeze on to your porridge.

Whilst chemically speaking, there's no fundamental difference between these different sources of sugar, the ones that you find naturally in food come with other positive nutrients (like the vitamin C and fibre you find in most fruit). Whereas adding sugar doesn't add any extra nutrients. So go easy when you're cooking.

Lots of the recipes in this book use honey, as we prefer this natural sugar made by bees. However, it's worth flagging that honey is still a type of sugar, meaning it's still high in calories. So when a recipe says a drizzle, it's just that. A drizzle. Not a drowning.

Regardless of where the sugars come from, when it comes to kids' teeth, it's all about how often and when you're eating sugars. The best way to maintain kids' dental health is to try (where possible) to keep sweet treats with meals. Have puddings, sweets and fruit after meals rather than in between. And keep the dentist onside by brushing twice daily with fluoride toothpaste.

As for the puds and sweet treats in this book, you can have pudding every day if you're just having a little bit. Think scoop rather than slop, a slice rather than a slab and one biscuit as opposed to the entire tin.

## Fats

All fats are high in calories, but the type of fat you use can make a difference. Fats can be grouped into 3 main types: saturated, polyunsaturated and monounsaturated. The more fats you can pick from the monounsaturated family the better as these are healthier fats. If you can't be faffed with checking labels every 5 minutes, go for olive- or rapeseed-oil based stuff. As for butter, use it sparingly rather than like tile adhesive.

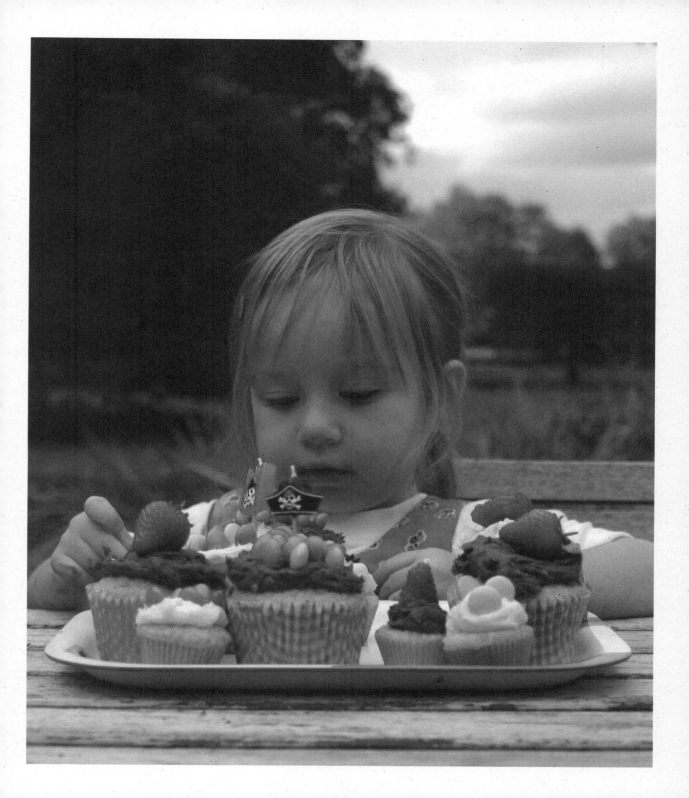

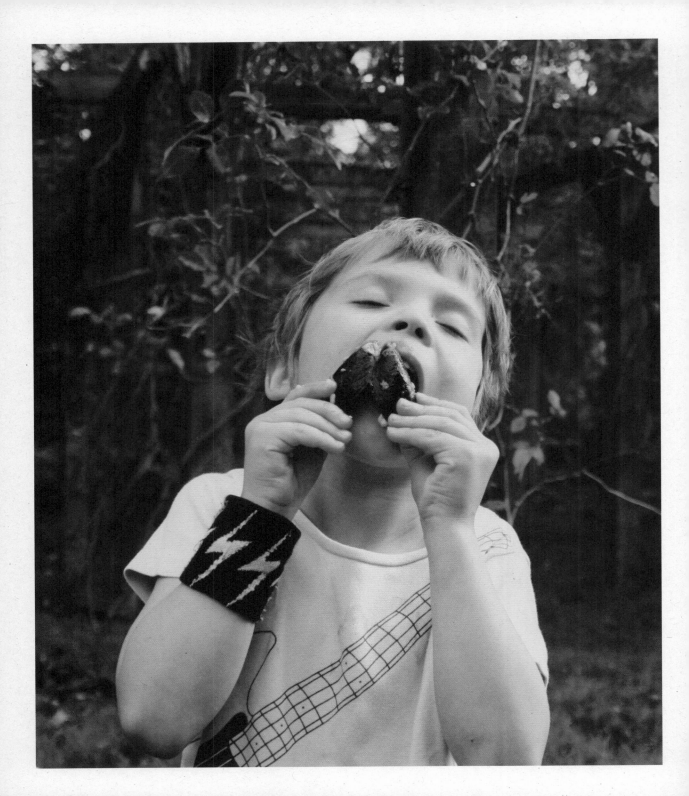

# A final word (before you start cooking)

As well as testing these recipes in our own kitchens, we've also had an army of mums, dads, kids, professional recipe writers and our own mums test these recipes before putting them in this book.

But everyone's kitchen scales work a little differently, no single oven is the same and there's always a way to make stuff better.

So if you have an easier way of doing something, a great tip to share or a nice addition to any of these recipes, we'd love to hear from you. Just drop us a line at wereallears@innocentdrinks.com and we'll try to add the changes to the next edition.

Ultimately, we hope that you enjoy everything in this book and use it a lot. Make the recipes, fill the pocket at the back and have a go at all the distractions and ideas for passing the time in between.

And if nothing else, think of it as a handy, book-shaped filing cabinet/multi-purpose home entertainment console that doesn't need batteries.

Happy cooking and eating.

love from innocent

REUSE AND reCYCLE.

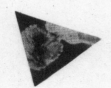

Recycling is not just that thing you do before you go to bed on a Tuesday. Making new stuff out of old stuff is really great. So as well as sorting out all your old papers, plastic and cans for the binman and making the weekly trip down the bottle bank, here's a few ways to make more out of what you've already got:

 **Buy one tote bag.** Put it in your handbag/coat pocket. Never leave the house without it. Never use a plastic bag again. Already got loads of plastic bags? Use them instead of bin liners and get fit putting the rubbish out every night.

 **Old laddered tights just about to go in the bin?** Store your potatoes in them. They like living in hosiery. Nobody knows why. Sam said his Nan knew, but we think she was just after some attention.

 **T-shirt seen better days?** Turn it into a cleaning rag and remember the days of youth every time you clean the bathroom.

 **Just finished the marmalade?** Keep old jam jars for storing stuff like dried lentils, buttons and bits of string.

 **Save all cartons with lids for leftover everything.** Designate a drawer in your kitchen to storing all your recycled, er, storage.

 **Stray buttons all over the place?** Keep them in a jar and sew onto your clothes at random whenever you lose a button, simultaneously customising your wardrobe and making you appear more interesting.

 **Save nice bits of newspaper for wrapping birthday presents.** Better still, carefully unwrap all the birthday and Christmas presents you receive this year, give the paper an iron and then reuse to wrap everyone's pressies next year.

 **Dry your teabags** on the radiator for endless cups of tea.

 **Use old orange peel** to keep next door's cat off your begonias.

 **Make presents** out of old toilet roll tubes.

 **Save the washing up and do it all in one go.** You'll save water, and be able to sneak your frying pan in with other people's stuff.

 **Have a shower with someone else.** Much less water and much more fun.

 **Save your cereal boxes** and make them into magazine/very important document holders. Never lose the car's MOT certificate again.

 **Bored of getting endless menus** and leaflets about estate agents' opening parties? Design yourself a smart new 'No junk mail please' sticker for your letter box.

# GOOD THINGS TO HAVE FOR

# BREAKFAST

# 101 things to do with eggs*

Eggs are brilliant. Nature's fragile portable packets of versatile genius. Or something like that. This section might feel a bit like that old phrase regarding said wonderfoods and your nan but there's nothing worse than getting your soldiers buttered and ready for action only to realise you've over-boiled your egg.

# THE GOOD EGG TEST

How to tell if your egg is fresh. Pop it into a glass of water and observe.

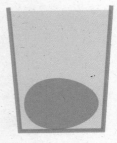

If it sinks to the bottom and stays there, it's good to go.

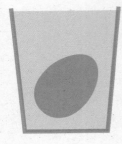

If it sinks but then floats at an angle, it's about a week old.

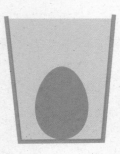

If it sinks and stands up, it's 2 weeks old.

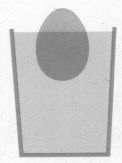

If it floats, bin it. Bad egg.

*Well, 15 or so.

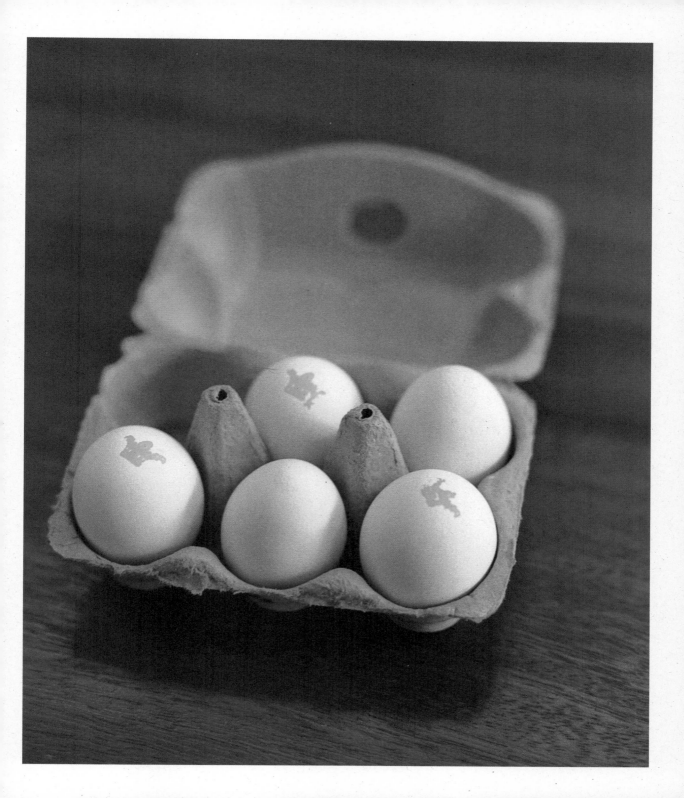

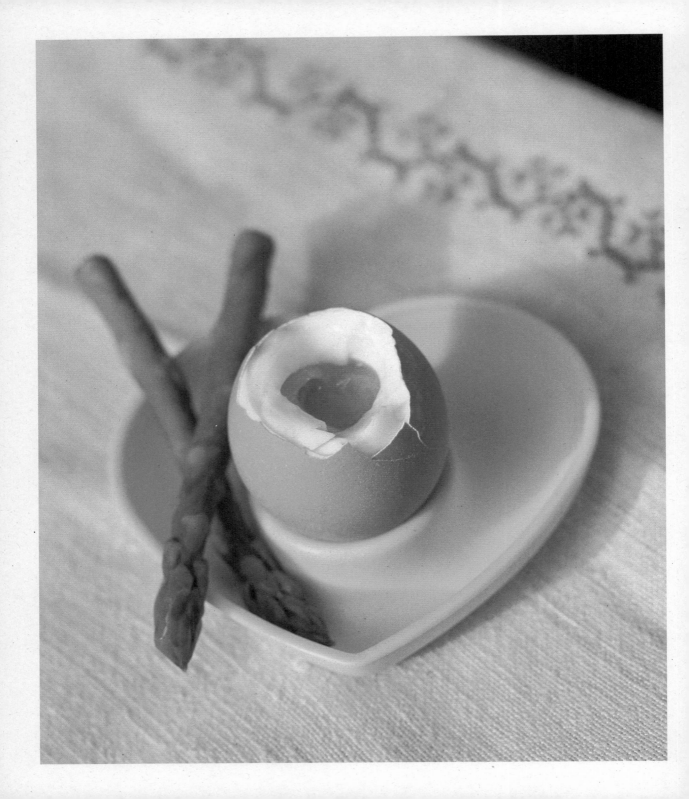

## Five foolproof egg tips

1. Boiling your eggs? The secret is using cold water and timing the eggs from the moment the water starts boiling.

2. Or get one of those egg-perfect egg timer things that changes colour to show you how runny your egg is. Available in all posh department stores and good cook shops.

3. Scrambling? Add a splash of milk and use a heavy-bottomed pan over a low heat with a wooden spoon for best results.

4. Don't have a fancy egg poacher? Just add a splash of vinegar to a pan of boiling water, crack in your eggs and simmer for 4 minutes.

5. Frying? Melt a knob of butter and a drizzle of olive oil, crack your eggs in and let them sit a minute for the white to set. Then spoon the hot butter or oil over the yolks. 2 minutes max.

## Good stuff to

### Dip in your eggs
- Buttered granary soldiers
- Asparagus spears if you're posh (5 spears = 1 of your 5-a-day)
- Fingers

### Scramble with your eggs
- Chopped herbs like chives, parsley and basil. If you like it spicy, sprinkle in a little curry powder, ground cumin or a chopped chilli.
- Spring onions (8 spring onions tick off 1 of your 5-a-day).
- Smoked salmon.
- Just before your eggs are fully cooked, add grated Cheddar.

### Serve with poached eggs
- Spinach
- Smoked haddock
- Good quality ham

# THINGS TO DO IN  **5** Minutes

While you're waiting for things to simmer

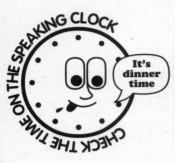

CHECK THE TIME ON THE SPEAKING CLOCK

It's dinner time

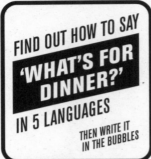

FIND OUT HOW TO SAY 'WHAT'S FOR DINNER?' IN 5 LANGUAGES

THEN WRITE IT IN THE BUBBLES

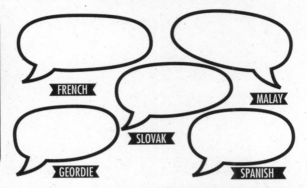

FRENCH

MALAY

SLOVAK

GEORDIE

SPANISH

---

**FIND 5 BLUE THINGS IN THE HOUSE. IF YOU CAN'T DO IT IN 5 MINUTES YOU HAVE TO WASH UP**

---

RUN UP AND DOWN THE STAIRS

Sharpen all the pencils you can find

GO AND CHECK THERE'S A GOOD SUPPLY OF LOO ROLL

TAKE A PHOTO

play YOUR FAVOURITE songs

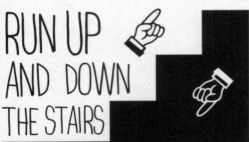

SEPARATE YOUR WHITES AND COLOURS

BALL UP YOUR SOCKS

DANCE UNTIL IT STOPS

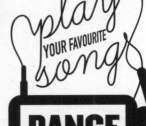

WALK LIKE AN EGYPTIAN, ALL THE WAY TO THE KITCHEN

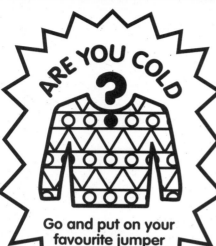

ARE YOU COLD ?

Go and put on your favourite jumper

START WRITING YOUR XMAS LIST (IT'S NEVER TOO EARLY)

INVENT YOUR IDEAL PET, DRAW IT, NAME IT AND TAKE IT FOR A WALK IN YOUR POCKET

GO AND BRUSH YOUR TEETH

GO ONLINE, FIND OUT WHICH FAMOUS PERSON'S BIRTHDAY IT IS AND SING THEM HAPPY BIRTHDAY

HOW MANY DIFFERENT LEAVES CAN YOU FIND IN YOUR GARDEN

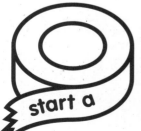

start a

masking

tape

message

THROW ALL THE RUBBISH OUT OF YOUR CAR

NIP NEXT DOOR FOR A CUP OF SUGAR

EVEN IF YOU DON'T NEED ONE

**START A RUMOUR. NOT TOO VICIOUS, MIND**

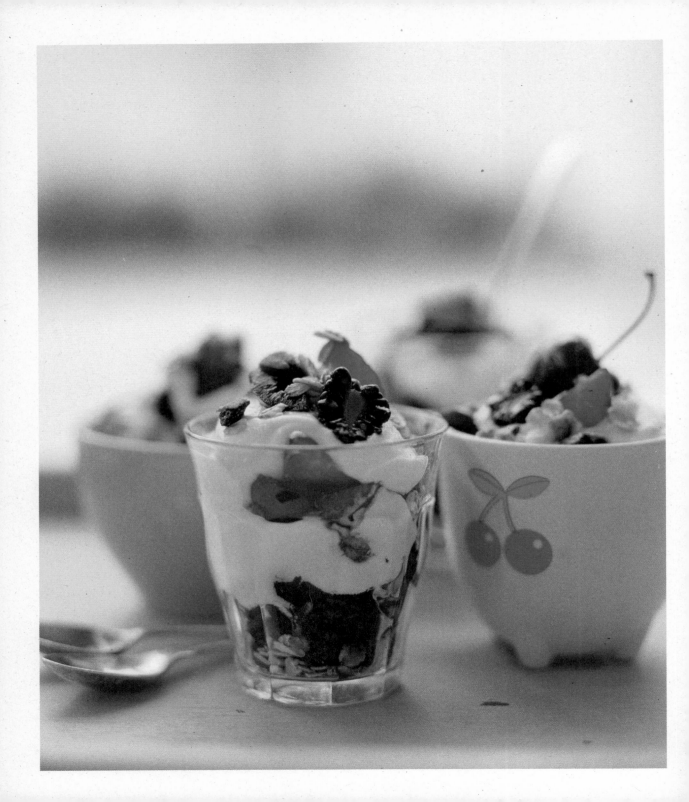

# Fun fruit for breakfast

Here are some quick ideas to get more fruit into your first meal of the day. All these recipes serve 1.

### Breakfast sundaes

**Pudding for breakfast, anyone? Thought so.**

Pop a handful of chopped fruit or berries into a glass or pot, spoon on 3 tablespoons of plain or fruit yoghurt, sprinkle with 2 tablespoons of oaty cereal or muesli. Eat with a teaspoon for a posh way to tick off 1 portion of your 5-a-day.

### Breakfast mash-up

**Much more fun than tipping one corner into another.**

Get a pudding bowl. Half-fill it with plain yoghurt. Chuck in a mixture of fruit that squashes well – strawberries, raspberries, blackberries, blueberries, bananas and peaches are all great. Drizzle with honey if required. Mash away.

### Blend it

**You can squeeze in loads of fruit by making your own smoothies and juices.**

You might even be able to squeeze in a sneaky carrot. Have a look at our smoothies and drinks section (see pages 316 to 345) for loads more ideas on getting fruit fast.

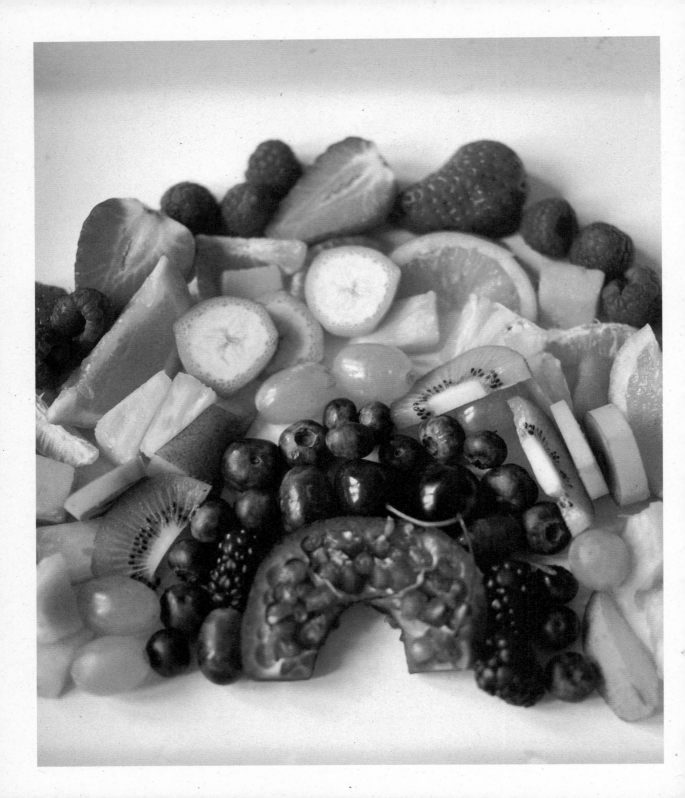

## Rainbow fruit salad

**Eat the rainbow. Literally.**

Get your kids to choose their favourite coloured fruit from each of the rainbow stripes opposite and build a rainbow on their plate.

Rules are you must have one of each colour. You don't have to follow the official rainbow mnemonic unless you really want to.* Just as long as you can eat the whole spectrum.

## Dippers

**The breakfast equivalent of the cheese fondue. Just with yoghurt and fruit as opposed to stale baguette and winey cheese.**

Drizzle a pot of plain yoghurt with honey and pop it on to a plate. Slice some fruit and artfully arrange around the pot. Allow dipping to commence.

Mangoes, melons, papayas, apples, pears and bananas work really well here as do satsuma and clementine segments. Or you could try popping grapes and strawberries on to cocktail sticks for slightly more advanced dipping.

* You know the one – *Richard of York gave blueberries in vain.*

# Toasty goodness

Toast is quick but jam is sugary, so here are a few ideas to liven up dough-based breakfasts. All these recipes serve 1.

## Hot banana sandwich

Mash up 1 banana in a bowl. Toast 2 slices of granary or wholemeal bread, spread the banana on top of one slice and drizzle with honey. Top with the other slice.

Or try spreading some peanut butter on your toast before spreading your banana on top. This counts as 1 portion of your 5-a-day.

## Breakfast crumpets

**Buck the teatime trend and kick off your day the crumpet way.**

Beat 1 egg in a shallow bowl. Dip 2 crumpets in and fry in a tiny bit of melted butter until golden. Then top with:

### Sweet
Serve with some honey, mashed-up berries and a blob of crème fraîche.

### Savoury
Cook some spinach or mushrooms in a knob of butter until wilted and soft and serve on top of your crumpets with a sprinkling of grated Cheddar cheese.

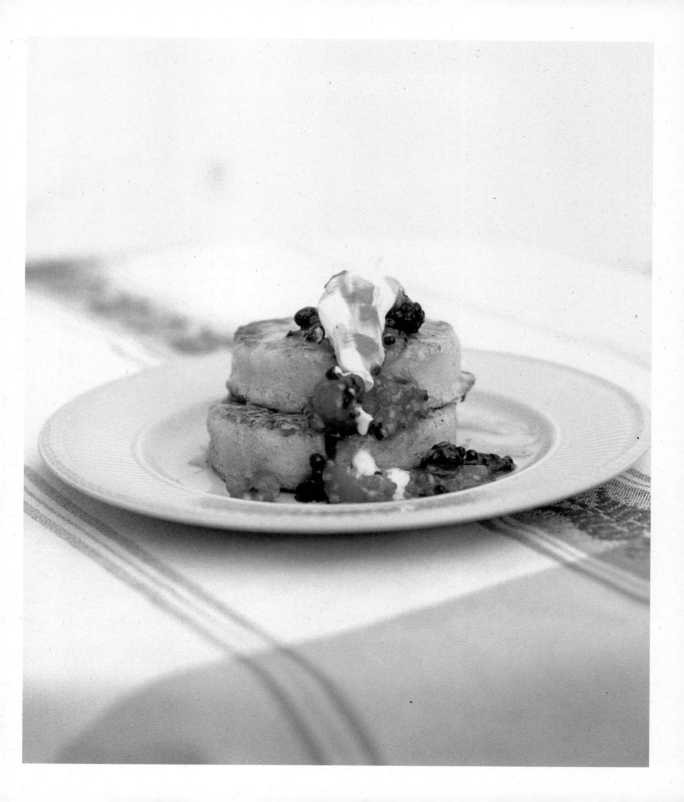

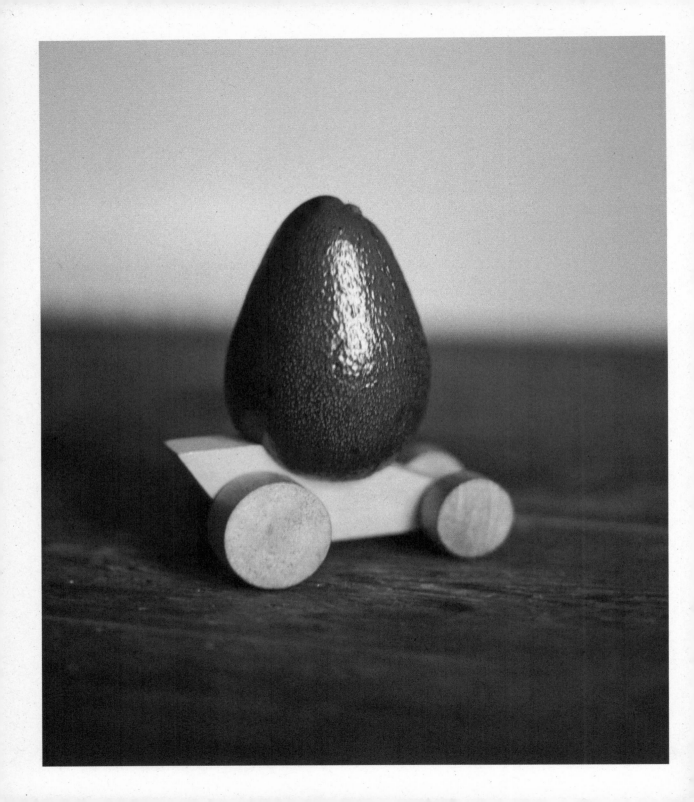

### Avocado to go

**Savoury breakfast made speedy.**

Mash up ½ an avocado in a bowl. Then finely dice 1 tomato and mix in another bowl with a splash of balsamic vinegar. Next, toast 1 slice of rye bread, spread on the mashed avocado and top with the chopped tomatoes. This counts as 2 portions of your 5-a-day.

### Toastie surprise

**This is dead easy to do in a toastie maker. If you don't have one, just use that good old-fashioned toaster-and-grill combo.**

Get 2 slices of granary or wholemeal bread and pop 1 slice in your toastie maker.

Add a handful of spinach, a sprinkling of grated Cheddar and carefully crack the egg into the centre.

Then place the other slice of bread on top and toast for a couple of minutes until golden. This counts as 1 portion of your 5-a-day.

### Muffin stack

**Pile 'em high and then gobble it all up.**

Split 1 English muffin in half and toast on both sides. Then layer up with a slice of Cheddar cheese, a slice of ham, a handful of fresh spinach and 1 sliced tomato for a tidy breakfast sandwich. This counts as 2 portions of your 5-a-day.

### Bake your own

Have a look at the 'Make and Bake' section on page 278 for some quick recipes on how to make your own bread and other doughy treats.

# Bear food

Some bears are big. Some bears are small. Some bears like to have their porridge plain. Others like to add berries, honey, nuts, fruit, seeds, brown sugar, jam, whatever-is-in-the-cupboard. So here's a standard porridge recipe and some ideas to try out. You can use milk, water, soya milk, rice milk, almond milk or apple juice for the liquid. And if you can't eat oats or just fancy a change, quinoa or millet flakes work really well as alternatives. All these recipes count as 1 portion of your 5-a-day, apart from Basic and Fancy.

Serves 1
½ a mug or a small handful
of oats
1 mug of milk, water, rice milk
or whatever you've got
handy

### Basic bear food
Put your oats into a pan, add your liquid and cook for a couple of minutes over a low heat, stirring to stop anything sticking. Once it's looking creamy, serve with your own toppings, or try one of these:

### Jungle bear
Make your porridge with milk or water, then add a mashed banana and a couple of tablespoons of desiccated coconut.

### Pink bear
Make your porridge with apple juice or water, then add a handful of strawberries or raspberries (fresh or frozen, depending on the time of year) and mash the berries in.

### Proper bear
Make your porridge with milk or water, then add chopped dried apricots, poppy seeds and a generous dollop of honey.

### Brown bear
Make your porridge with milk or water, then add a handful of raisins, a pinch of cinnamon and a swirl of maple syrup.

### Fancy bear
Make your porridge with apple juice or soya milk, or half of each, then grate in half an apple and mix well.

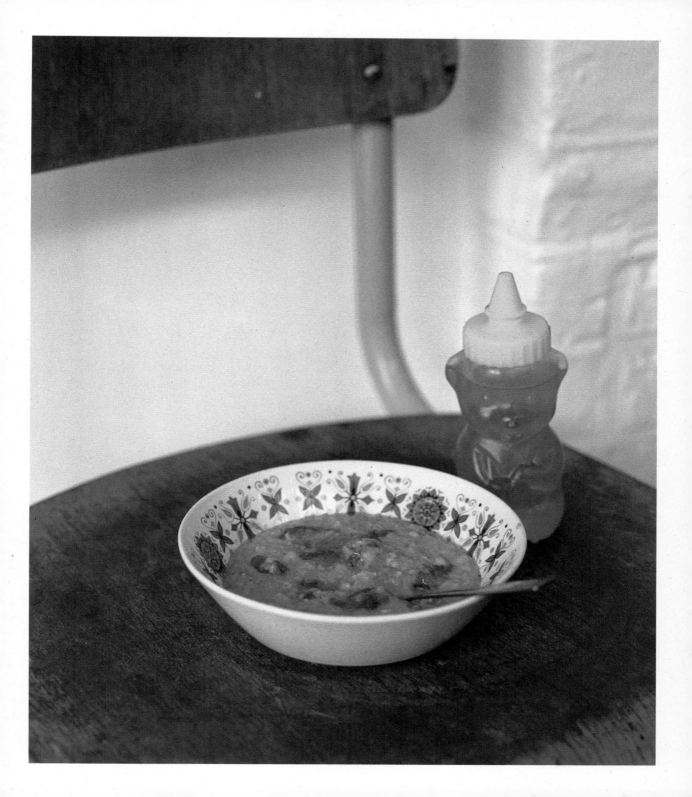

# Bubble and squeak

Cockney rhyming slang for week, and also a great way to use up roasted or leftover veg (sounds far more exciting than medium-sized circles of refried cabbage and spud).

Preheat your oven to 180°C/350°F/gas mark 4.

Bring a large pan of water to the boil. Add the potatoes and root vegetables and boil until tender. Meanwhile, in another pan, cook the cabbage in boiling water for about 5 minutes, until wilted.

Drain both pans into a large colander and allow the veg to steam for a couple of minutes. Then mash them together with a fork, leaving a few chunky bits here and there.

Pop your sausages on a baking tray and bake in the oven for 30 minutes, remembering to turn them from time to time until golden.

While they're baking, heat a couple of knobs of butter in a big frying pan and fry the leek until soft. Add the thyme and the mashed veg and mix well, then sprinkle in the cheese.

Remove the mixture from the pan to a board and divide into 4 portions, then mould each one into a flat cake - or 2 smaller ones for the kids.

Return the frying pan to the heat, add a couple more knobs of butter and lightly fry the cakes on both sides until golden brown.

Serve the bubble and squeak cakes with the sausages and a generous dollop of traffic-light ketchup (page 310) or tomato purée mixed with balsamic vinegar or Worcestershire sauce.

Serves 4
1½ portions of your 5-a-day

300g floury potatoes, peeled and cut into chunks
300g root vegetables (sweet potatoes, parsnips, turnips, swedes and so on), peeled and cut into chunks
½ a green cabbage, shredded
6 good-quality sausages
a few knobs of butter
1 large leek, washed and finely chopped
a few sprigs of thyme, stalks removed
100g Cheddar cheese, coarsely grated

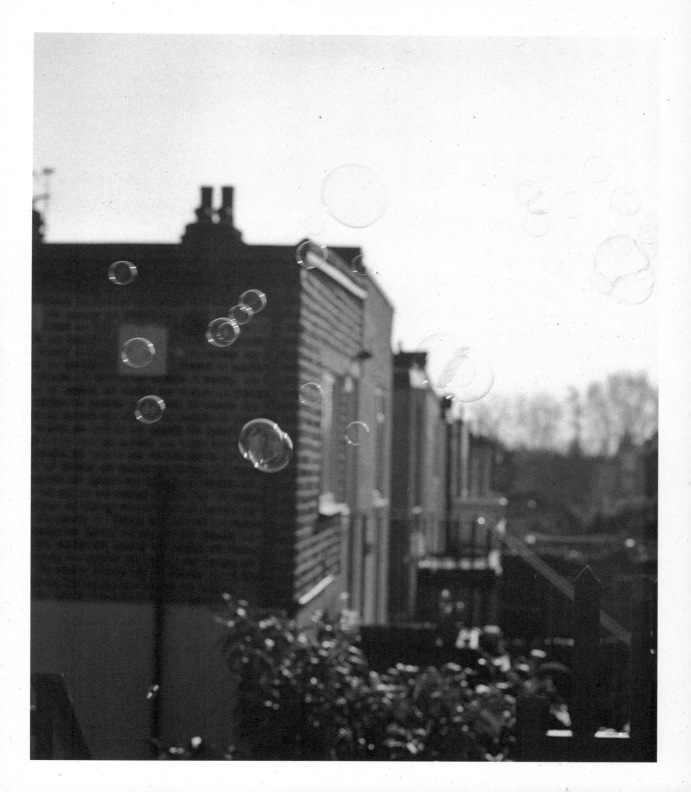

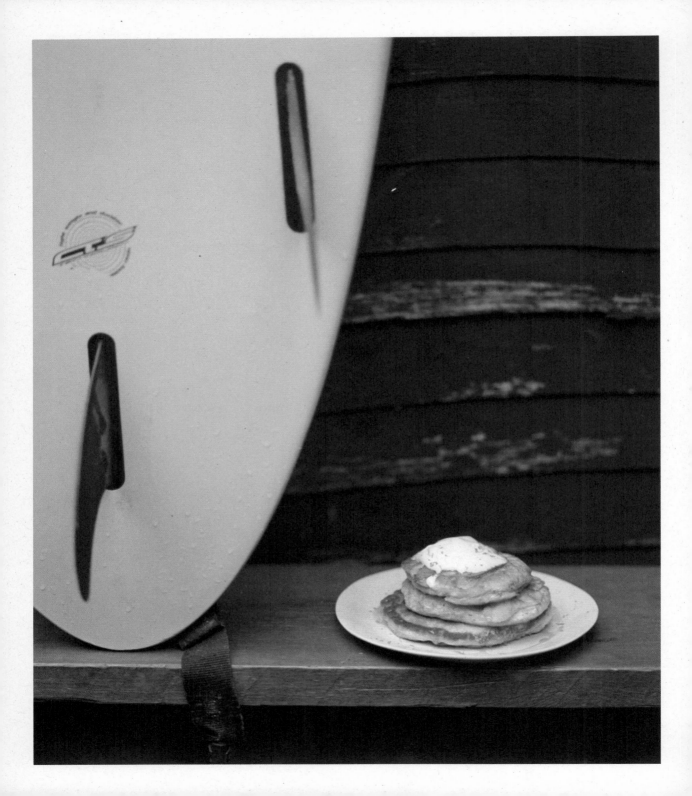

# Surfer's pancakes

The raddest way to start the day. But before you hit the waves, don't forget to pack a warm jumper, a flask of tea and a hot water bottle to warm up your towel. Post-dip chill doth not an enjoyable breakfast make.

Makes 12 pancakes
counts towards your 5-a-day

2 large free-range eggs
1 mug of plain flour
a handful of oats
1 teaspoon baking powder
a pinch of salt
1 mug of milk
butter, for frying
2 bananas, halved widthways
   then sliced thinly lengthways

To serve
honey or maple syrup
1 lime
crème fraîche (optional)

Preheat your oven to 120°C/250°F/gas mark 1 so that you can keep your pancakes warm.

Separate the eggs, putting the yolks into one bowl and the whites into another. Add the flour, oats, baking powder and salt to the yolks, then pour in the milk and mix well to remove any lumps.

Now whisk the egg whites until they form firm peaks and gently fold them into the pancake batter. Don't over-mix or you'll get flat pancakes.

Melt some butter in a medium non-stick frying pan over a medium heat and then add a couple of ladles of batter. Allow to settle for a minute, then lay a couple of banana slices across the pancake and cook until bubbles start to rise.

Once the bottom of the pancake is golden, flip it over using a fish slice and cook until the other side is golden brown. Pop it on to a plate, cover with foil and place in the oven to keep warm while you get on with making the rest of your pancakes. To speed things up a bit, you could have 2 pans on the go, one big and one small.

Serve the pancakes drizzled with honey or maple syrup, and a squeeze of fresh lime juice, a blob of crème fraîche, if using, and a scattering of lime zest.

If you don't fancy bananas, try using sliced fresh mango, raspberries, blueberries, or a mixture of all these instead. Tinned peaches in their own juice also work really well here.

# Breakfast burritos

Burrito is Spanish for 'little donkey'. There are no donkeys in this recipe.

Serves 4 (2 big people and 2 small ones)

1½ portions of your 5-a-day

4 soft tortilla wraps
a dash of olive oil
1 red chilli, deseeded and finely chopped
1 spring onion, finely chopped
1 garlic clove, peeled and finely chopped
1 x 400g tin of borlotti or cannellini beans, drained and rinsed
a handful of cherry tomatoes, halved
1 avocado
juice and grated zest of 1 lime
a bunch of coriander, roughly chopped, stalks and all
a knob of butter
6 free-range eggs, well beaten
100g Cheddar or Manchego cheese, grated

Preheat your oven to 150°C/300°F/gas mark 2. Wrap your tortillas in greaseproof paper and place them in the oven to warm through.

Put a dash of olive oil in a pan. Add the chilli, spring onion and garlic and fry until the garlic starts to brown. Add the beans and half the tomatoes and simmer over a very low heat while you make the guacamole.

Finely dice the rest of the tomatoes and put into a bowl. Halve the avocado, remove the stone and scoop the flesh into the bowl. Add the juice of the lime and half the grated zest, season and mix together.

Add half the chopped coriander to the bean mix and remove from the heat. Add the other half to the guacamole.

Melt the butter in a non-stick saucepan and add the beaten eggs. Allow them to settle in the pan for 30 seconds or so, then, using a wooden spoon, gently fold the eggs as they cook until they are cooked to your desired consistency.

Once the eggs are cooked, take the warm tortillas out of the oven and place one on each serving plate. Add a generous serving of beans to each tortilla.

Top the bean mix with a big scoop of scrambled eggs, a heaped tablespoon of guacamole and a liberal sprinkling of grated cheese. Roll up the tortilla and serve.

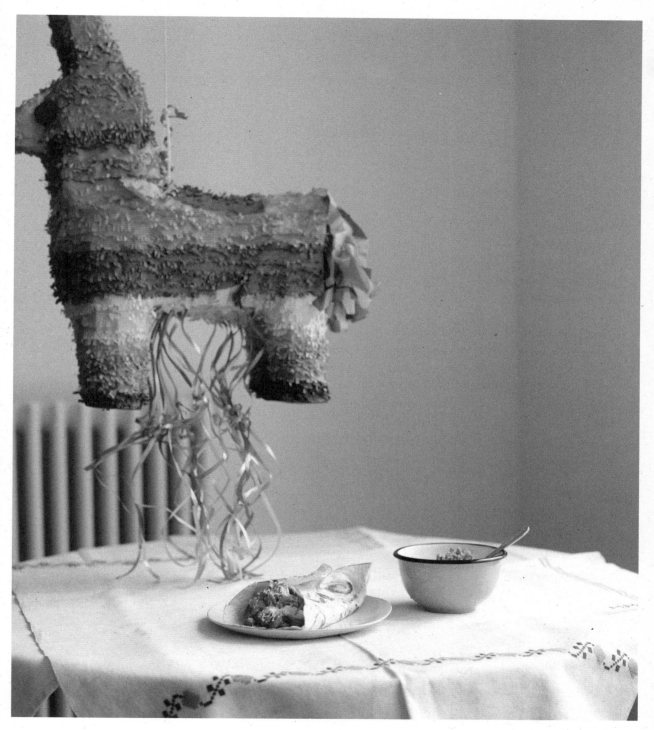

'I beg your pardon. I think you'll find I'm actually a hovering piñata.'

# French toast fingers

*'Mince alors, ce n'est pas un toast à la française ça, juste du pain perdu qui frime. Dès la fin du petit déjeuner, j'appellerai moi-même Monsieur l'ambassadeur pour déposer un rapport. Bon, et maintenant où ai-je mis le sirop d'érable?'\**

Serves 4

counts towards your 5-a-day

2 free-range eggs
a splash of milk
1 tablespoon sugar
4 thick slices of granary/
   brown bread
a knob of butter
a couple of handfuls of
   blueberries or other
   seasonal fruit
maple syrup or honey, for
   drizzling
plain yoghurt or crème fraîche

Preheat your oven to 150°C/300°F/gas mark 2.

Crack your eggs into a bowl, add the milk and sugar and mix well.

Cut the bread into chunky fingers and dip them one at a time into the eggy mixture, making sure they're thoroughly coated.

Melt some butter in a non-stick frying pan over a medium heat and quickly fry the eggy fingers (4 at a time) for a minute or so on each side, until golden brown. Put them on to a plate, cover them with foil and pop them into the oven to keep warm while you make the rest of the fingers.

To speed things up, get a helper to dip the fingers or have 2 pans on the go.

Once all the fingers are cooked, serve topped with blueberries, a drizzle of maple syrup or honey and a dollop of plain yoghurt or crème fraîche.

Try using berries in the summer and stewed plums and apples in the winter. See page 256 for some ideas.

*\*'Oh my gosh. This is not French toast. This is just eggy bread that's got too big for its boots. I'm going to call the Ambassador right after breakfast and report this to him myself. Now, where did I put the maple syrup?'*

# Spanish eggs-in-a-pot

**Think of this breakfast as more in-a-cobbled-courtyard-overlooking-the-Andalucian-hills than noisy-all-you-can-eat-full-English-on-the-Costa-del-Sol-post-sunlounger-bagsying.**

Serves 4

1 portion of your 5-a-day

2 fresh chorizo sausages, diced

4 spring onions, trimmed and finely sliced

3 big handfuls of spinach, washed and roughly chopped

1 small jar of roasted red peppers, drained and chopped

8 cherry tomatoes, quartered

4 free-range eggs

a pinch of smoked paprika

Preheat your oven to 180°C/350°F/gas mark 4.

Fry the diced chorizo and spring onions in a large dry frying pan for about 10 minutes, until crispy.

Add the spinach with 1 tablespoon of water and allow to wilt.

Divide the mixture between 4 ramekins, adding the peppers and tomatoes, and give everything a good stir.

Crack an egg into each pot, season with salt and pepper and a pinch of smoked paprika and pop into the oven for about 15 to 20 minutes, until the eggs are just set.

Serve with a good hunk of granary bread.

# SUNDAY NIGHT IS ALRIGHT

Sunday blues getting you down?
Feeling a bit miffed that you've
got to go to work/school tomorrow?
Don't get crabby, get chipper and
reclaim Sunday as Funday using
the handy guide opposite.

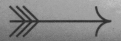

# THE 30 STEPS TO SUNDAY HEAVEN

1. Have a lie in
2. Or if the kids wake you up, stick an 'educational' DVD on downstairs (Toy Story)
3. Continue lie in for a further 23 minutes
4. Get up
5. Stroll to paper shop in dressing gown (dog optional)
6. Papers + coffee + croissants or last night's leftover fish pie (see page 146)
7. Wash (maybe)
8. Get the roast on (see page 188)
9. Take kids to park/garden centre/watch Toy Story 2
10. Walk home
11. Get the roast on the table
12. Tuck in
13. Wash up
14. Snooze
15. Check football scores
16. Read a bit more of the paper
17. Dog walk
18. Start baking (see page 278)
19. Sort the recycling
20. Clean your shoes
21. Make tomorrow's packed lunch (see page 76)
22. Sample the fruits of your baking labour
23. Settle down to watch Sunday film (Toy Story 3)
24. Run the bath
25. Sunday night hair wash for the little ones
26. Put kids to bed
27. Eat Sunday roast leftover sandwich
28. Watch costume drama
29. Doze off on sofa
30. Put yourself to bed

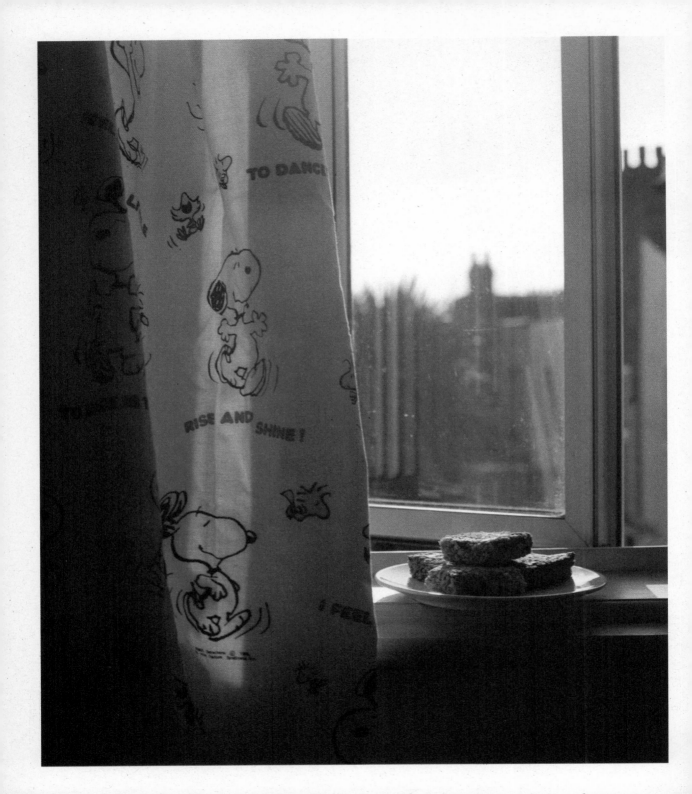

# Rise and shine flapjacks

**Slept in? Running late? Out of milk? Fear not. This is the on-the-go breakfast saviour. Perfect for mornings that don't quite go according to plan.**

Makes about 12 flapjacks
counts towards your 5-a-day

a handful of dried apricots
a large handful of stoned
  dates
150g butter
3 tablespoons apple juice
3 tablespoons runny honey
225g porridge oats
a handful of dried fruit
  (raisins, sour cherries,
  cranberries, whatever you
  fancy)
2 tablespoons unsweetened
  desiccated coconut

Preheat your oven to 150°C/300°F/gas mark 2 and lightly grease a 20 x 30cm baking tray.

Chop the apricots and dates as small as you can, as these will help the flapjacks stick together.

Melt the butter in a small pan, then take off the heat and add the apple juice and honey.

Put the chopped fruit and the rest of the ingredients into a big bowl. Pour over the butter mixture and mix together with a wooden spoon.

Spread the mixture out on the baking tray and bake in the oven for 25 minutes, until golden brown.

Allow to cool for 15 minutes, then cut into bars and store in an airtight container – they will keep for up to a week.

# Make-your-own muesli

Ferreting out all the bits of muesli you don't like is a joyless task. Far better to make your own, enjoy your breakfast and use those precious regained minutes to perfect your Standing Mountain Pose.

Preheat your oven to 180°C/350°F/gas mark 4.

Put the oats, chopped nuts and seeds into a deep baking tray. Drizzle with honey and the cinnamon and give everything a good stir.

Bake in the oven for 12 to 15 minutes, giving the tray a good shake halfway through.

Once it's all looking toasty, take it out of the oven, add the coconut and the dried fruit and give it another stir.

Pop it back into the oven for about 5 minutes, until the fruit becomes soft and gooey.

Allow to cool completely, then store in an airtight container. It'll keep for up to 4 weeks. Have it with milk, yoghurt or fresh fruit, use for breakfast sundaes (page 37) or simply have a handful as a healthy snack.

Makes a big jar
(enough for 10 breakfasts)
counts towards your 5-a-day

6 handfuls of rolled oats
a handful of pecans, roughly chopped
a handful of pumpkin seeds
a handful of sunflower seeds
2 tablespoons runny honey
a pinch of ground cinnamon
2 tablespoons unsweetened desiccated coconut
2 handfuls of your favourite dried fruit (golden raisins, sour cherries, chopped dates, chopped apricots, cranberries, blueberries, whatever you fancy)

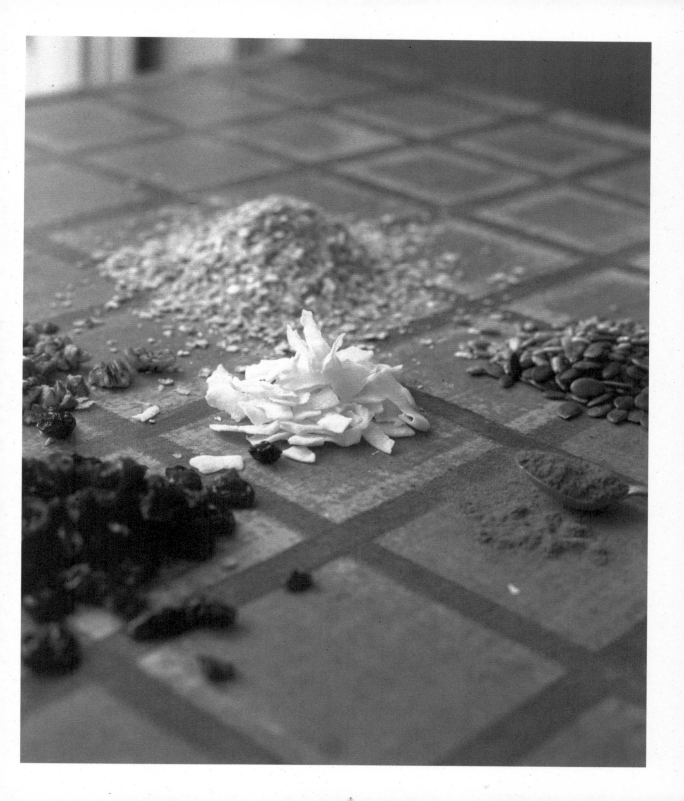

# Banana and bran flake muffins

Last out of the fruit bowl, first in the bin and blamed for many a fruit fly gathering, brown bananas get a rough ride. So allow the ripe, the brown and the downright speckly to redeem themselves in this recipe. Unless you happen to be partial to hosting an insect disco.

100g unsalted butter
2 tablespoons runny honey
3 ripe bananas
2 large free-range eggs
125ml milk
100g bran flakes, crushed
200g self-raising flour
100g porridge oats
a big handful of raisins

Preheat your oven to 180°C/350°F/gas mark 4 and place 12 muffin cases in a muffin tray.

Melt the butter and honey in a saucepan and remove from the heat.

Peel the bananas and mash them in a big bowl. Add the eggs and milk and whisk together.

Put the bran flakes into a sandwich bag and give them a good bash with a rolling pin. Add to the banana mixture along with the flour, oats and raisins, and finally stir in the honey mixture.

Mix it all together but don't mix it too much. That's the trick to perfect muffins. Divide the mixture evenly between the muffin cases and pop them into the oven for 25 to 30 minutes, until golden brown.

The muffins will keep for up to a week, in an airtight container.

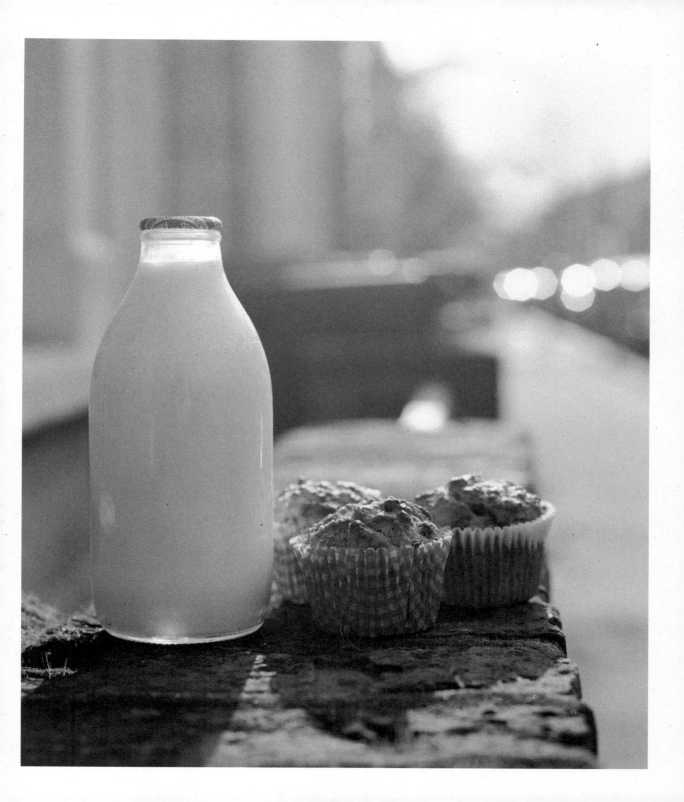

# GOOD THINGS TO HAVE FOR

---

# LUNCH

# Jacket potatoes

**An all-round lunchtime classic. Just respect the basic methods for baking your spud and then go wild with the toppings.**

First things first. Get a potato and prick all over with a fork. Then rub in a little bit of oil and salt and bake in the oven at 200°C/400°F/gas mark 6 for an hour or so till crispy on the outside, fluffy on the inside. If you're pushed for time, stick your spud in the microwave for 10 minutes on full power (turning over halfway through). Then rub in oil and salt and pop in the oven for 10 minutes to crisp up. Alternatively, give it the old oil and salt treatment, wrap in foil and pop on the campfire for 22 renditions of Gin gan gooli/that one about a pizza hut.

## Fillings

**Here are some ideas to fill your potato with once it's cooked:**

Flake 1 fillet of smoked mackerel (skin and bones removed) and mix with 2 chopped spring onions and 2 tablespoons of crème fraîche.

Mash 3 tablespoons of cooked peas with plain yoghurt and some chopped mint.

Chop up 2 cooked beetroots, add a handful of rocket, some crumbled goat's cheese and mix together with a sprinkling of fresh mint.

## Grillings

**For a less chilling filling, cut your cooked spud in half, top with one of the following and stick under the grill until bubbling:**

Snip up a grilled rasher of bacon and a handful of fresh spinach, sprinkle over your spud and top with some grated Cheddar cheese.

Chop up 2 sundried tomatoes, 4 stoned black olives, ½ a ball of mozzarella and sprinkle with a few basil leaves.

Stir 3 tablespoons of sweetcorn into ½ a tin of drained tuna and sprinkle with grated cheese.

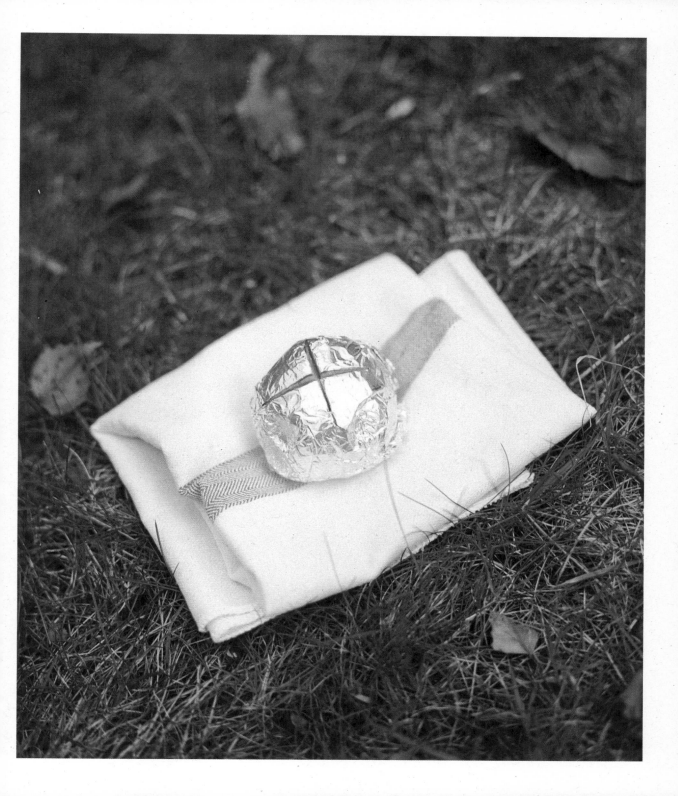

# Old bread and squashed tomato salad

Stale bread? Don't waste it on the ducks. Until ducks learn to say thank you, we're not giving them any more stale bread. Ducks – good at swimming, less good on manners. Buy your own ciabatta, Beakface.

Preheat your oven to 180°C/350°F/gas mark 4.

Slice the bigger tomatoes into a large salad bowl, squash in the smaller ones, and sprinkle with a couple of pinches of sea salt. Give it a stir and set aside.

If your bread is really stale you can skip the next bit. If it's still quite soft, put it on a baking tray and dry it out in the oven for about 10 minutes, until golden. Then allow to cool.

Add the garlic, peppers, olives and capers to the bowl of tomatoes and give everything a good mix. Tear up the basil leaves and add to the bowl, then add the olive oil and vinegar and toss everything together.

Taste to see if more seasoning is needed, then add the bread and give everything a jolly good mix.

Serves 4
2 portions of your 5-a-day

600g different-sized ripe tomatoes
a sprinkling of sea salt
300g ciabatta or sourdough bread (stale is best), ripped into chunks
1 garlic clove, peeled and finely chopped
4 roasted red peppers from a jar, roughly chopped
a handful of stoned black olives
a small handful of capers
a big bunch of basil
100ml olive oil
2 tablespoons red wine vinegar

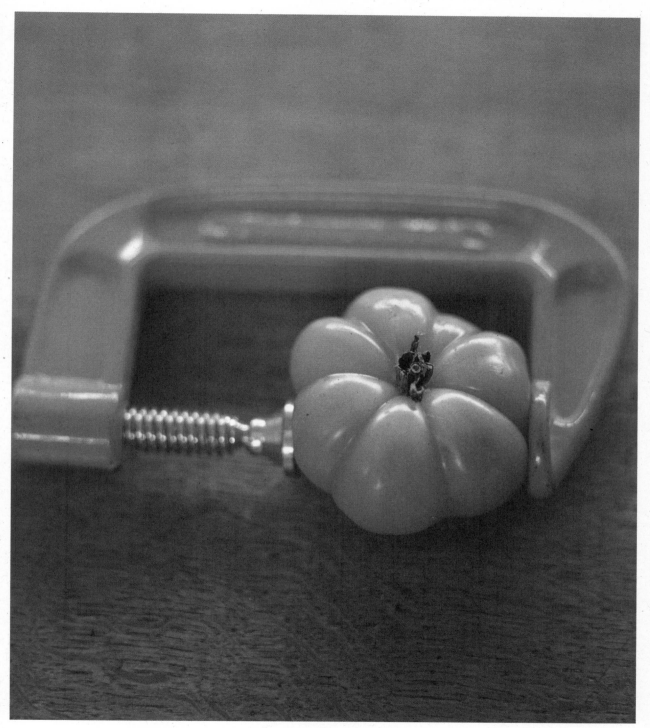

'I'll never tell you where the money's hidden.'

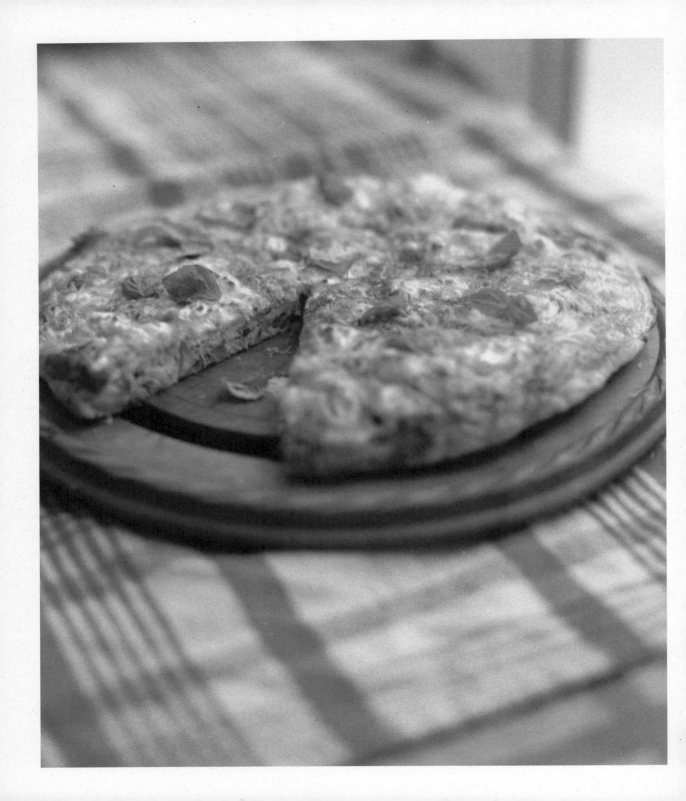

# Summer frittata

You can put almost anything you like in a frittata. Leftover cooked veg, grated cheese, sliced sausage, marmalade, saveloy, whelks, those little bags of complimentary peanuts ... whatever you like.

This is a recipe for summer but there's also a winter version at the bottom of the page. Feel free to improvise with anything you like, using the ingredients listed as your basis.

Serves 2 as a main,
4 as a snack
2 portions of your 5-a-day

4 courgettes, grated
2 handfuls of podded fresh
   broad beans
zest of 1 lemon
a small bunch of basil
a good grating of Parmesan
   cheese
4 free-range eggs, beaten
a bit of butter
1 small soft goat's cheese

First, heat your grill to medium.

Grate the courgettes into a bowl and sprinkle with a pinch of salt to allow the water to seep out. Leave to one side for a few minutes, then squeeze out the water with your hands and pour it away.

Put the grated courgettes back into the bowl and add the broad beans. Make sure you remove the bright green beans from their pale tough outer skins first. Add the lemon zest and tear in some basil. Add the grated Parmesan and the eggs and mix together well.

In a medium frying pan, heat a small knob of butter till it bubbles and pour in the frittata mixture.

Dot the top with little blobs of goat's cheese and cook on a low heat for 5 to 10 minutes, until the bottom is golden brown.

Finally, pop the whole thing under the grill until the cheese is golden on top.

Scatter with basil leaves and finally serve in slices, with a green salad and some wholemeal pitta bread.

## Winter frittata
During the colder months, replace the grated courgettes with 4 cooked beetroots, chopped into small chunks, and use a little bit of dill instead of the basil. Try to go for the unvinegary type of beetroot if you can.

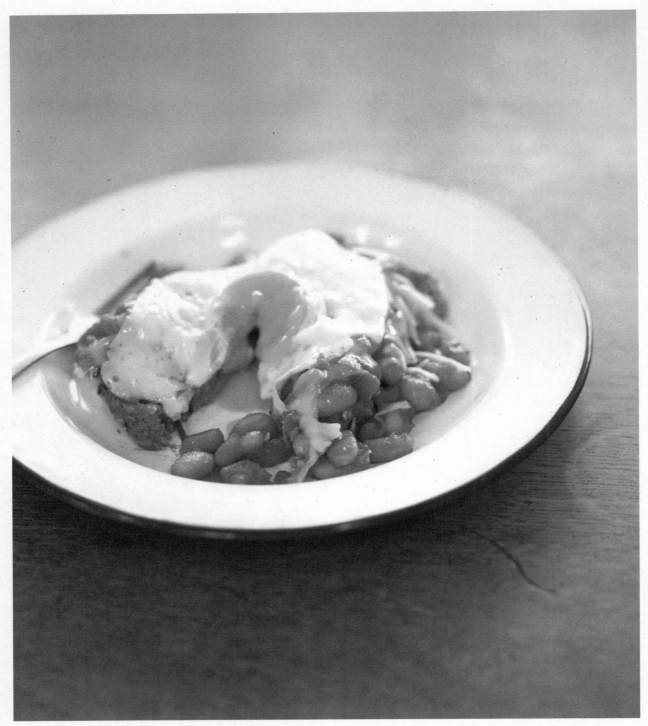

Fine dining by way of a tin opener.

# Homemade beans on toast

There are lots of ditties about beans involving words that rhyme with 'heart' but, in this instance, beans means toast. And smoked paprika and garlic and a sprig or two of rosemary.

Serves 4
2 portions of your 5-a-day

olive oil
1 red onion, peeled and finely chopped
1 garlic clove, peeled and crushed
a sprig of rosemary
1 teaspoon smoked paprika
2 x 400g tins of cannellini beans, drained and rinsed
1 x 400g tin of chopped tomatoes
a drizzle of balsamic vinegar
4 large free-range eggs
butter, for frying
4 slices of brown or granary bread

Heat a pan over a medium heat, add a little olive oil and fry the onion, garlic and rosemary for 5 minutes, or until the onion is soft.

Add the smoked paprika and cook for a further minute or so. Then tip in the drained beans and tomatoes and simmer for about 20 minutes, adding a little water if necessary.

Pick out the rosemary stalk, drizzle in some balsamic vinegar, season with salt and pepper and simmer for another 5 minutes, until the sauce has reduced.

Fry the eggs in a little butter and toast your bread.

Serve a good scoop of beans on each piece of toast, and top with a fried egg – you can add some grated Cheddar if you fancy it.

# Quick ricotta pancakes

We say yes to dogs in jumpers, yes to dancing with nans at weddings and yes to eating these pancakes on Wednesday afternoons in April, Thursday mornings in May or whenever you flipping well like.

**Serves 4**
1 portion of your 5-a-day

2 large free-range eggs
1 mug of milk
1 mug of plain flour
a pinch of salt
4 tablespoons ricotta cheese
a sprinkling of freshly grated
    nutmeg
butter, for cooking
4 big handfuls of spinach
1 lemon

Preheat your oven to its lowest heat, to keep your pancakes warm as you cook them.

Put the eggs, milk, flour and salt into a bowl and mix until you have a smooth batter. Add the ricotta and nutmeg and leave the batter to stand for about 15 minutes.

Heat a little butter in a large non-stick pan and spoon in a ladle of the batter, spreading it out a bit. Cook for a couple of minutes, until the pancake is golden underneath, then flip it over (using a fish slice if you're not confident at flipping) and cook on the other side.

Once your first pancake is cooked, pop it on to a plate, cover it with foil and stick it in the warm oven while you make the rest.

When all the pancakes are ready, melt some butter in a frying pan, add the spinach and allow it to wilt down for a few minutes, adding a splash of water if needed. Squeeze in the juice of half the lemon.

Serve the pancakes with a big pile of spinach and the remaining lemon half to squeeze over.

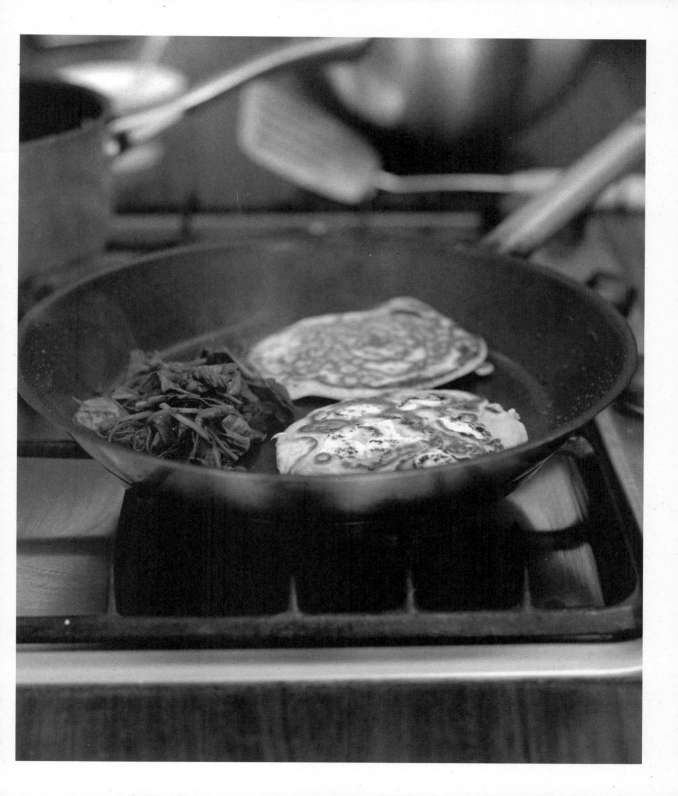

# THINGS TO DO IN 10 Minutes

While you're waiting for things to burn

## Sort out the recycling

Have a quick game of

# SNAP

Best of 5 wins

Make a new playlist

SEND PAPER AEROPLANE MESSAGES TO YOUR NEIGHBOURS

hello

USE A LEMON TO DO SOME CLEANING

GO AND HIDE IN THE GARDEN (REALLY WELL) AND GET A LITTLE PERSON TO FIND IT

PILLOW FIGHT

HIDE SECRET NOTES AROUND THE HOUSE...

# LEARN TO JUGGLE WITH TOMATOES

If you have any stale bread, break into beak size pieces for the ducks. Or use it to make the old bread and squashed tomato salad over on page 66

**PACK YOUR BAG FOR TOMORROW AND GET AN EXTRA 10 MINUTES IN BED IN THE MORNING**

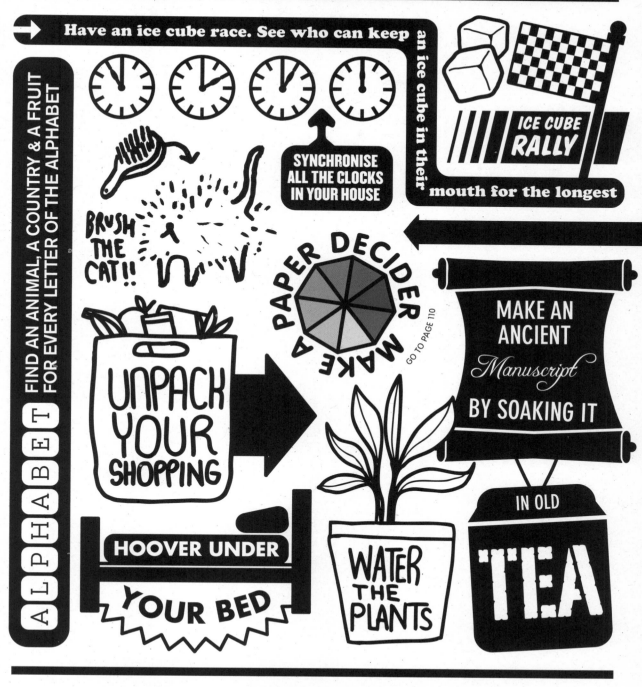

Have an ice cube race. See who can keep an ice cube in their mouth for the longest

ICE CUBE RALLY

SYNCHRONISE ALL THE CLOCKS IN YOUR HOUSE

BRUSH THE CAT!!

ALPHABET FIND AN ANIMAL, A COUNTRY & A FRUIT FOR EVERY LETTER OF THE ALPHABET

MAKE A PAPER DECIDER

GO TO PAGE 110

MAKE AN ANCIENT *Manuscript* BY SOAKING IT

IN OLD

TEA

UNPACK YOUR SHOPPING

HOOVER UNDER YOUR BED

WATER THE PLANTS

HAVE A STARING CONTEST ◉ ◉

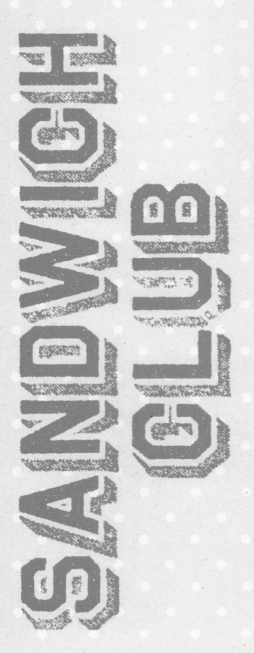

# SANDWICH CLUB

The recipe for a successful sandwich is relatively straightforward:
Take 2 bits of bread. Whack your favourite food between them. Cut in half. Eat.

Granted, this formula is a bit trickier if gravy, oysters or trifle are your food of choice. But as long as you cut the bread thick enough and wear a bib, you'll be fine. Here are some of our top sandwich fillings.

## HLTC

2 slices of good ham, a handful of shredded lettuce, 4 slices of cucumber and 1 medium tomato.

## POSH HLTC

2 slices of prosciutto, a handful of round lettuce, 7 cherry tomatoes, 4 slices of cucumber and some basil.

## CHEESE & TOMATO

A slice of Cheddar cheese topped with 1 sliced tomato or 7 cherry tomatoes.

## CHEESE & APPLE

Core and slice 1 apple. Then layer up with some Cheddar cheese.

## SWEET SWEET SLAW

Grate half an apple and half a carrot. Then finely chop 2 spring onions, add a teaspoon of mayo and a squeeze of lemon juice then mix with a little bit of grated cheese.

## THE GREEN ITALIAN

Spread 1 tablespoon of pea-green dip (page 106), add a handful of spinach, half a ball of torn up mozzarella and some fresh basil.

## EGG MAYO

Chop up 1 hard-boiled egg and 2 gherkins, mix in a handful of cress, a squeeze of salad cream and lemon juice and top with cracked black pepper.

## PRAWN COCKTAIL

Sprinkle a handful of cooked prawns over a handful of shredded cos lettuce, half a sliced avocado, a squeeze of lemon and some cracked black pepper.

## CHICKEN & AVOCADO

Pile up leftover roast chicken, half an avocado, a little drizzle of mayo and a squeeze of lemon juice.

## HUMMUS & CARROT

2 tablespoons of hummus (page 106), 1 grated carrot and a squeeze of lemon juice. Add raisins for a sweet treat.

## GOOD THINGS TO DO WITH CREAM CHEESE

Add it to half a grated courgette, a squeeze of lemon and cracked black pepper. Top with tomato, lettuce and a quarter of an avocado. Pile with salami or ham or top with some smoked salmon and a squeeze of lemon juice.

## MARMITE

Get some Marmite and some bread. Make into a sandwich. Rejoice or recoil.

## HANDHELD PICNIC

1 slice of good-quality ham, 1 slice of Cheddar cheese, a handful of shredded cos lettuce, 1 sliced tomato and a smidge of mustard.

## PEPPERED SALAMI

3 big slices of salami and 1 roasted red pepper from a jar.

## FRUIT AND NUT

1 tablespoon of peanut butter, half a sliced banana and 7 sliced strawberries.

## THE BREADED KING OF GREECE

Layer up a big handful of spinach, 1 sliced tomato, 6 slices of cucumber, some chopped olives and a little crumbled feta. For added Greekness, serve on a broken plate and dance about.

# • JOHN MONTAGU, WE SALUTE YOU •

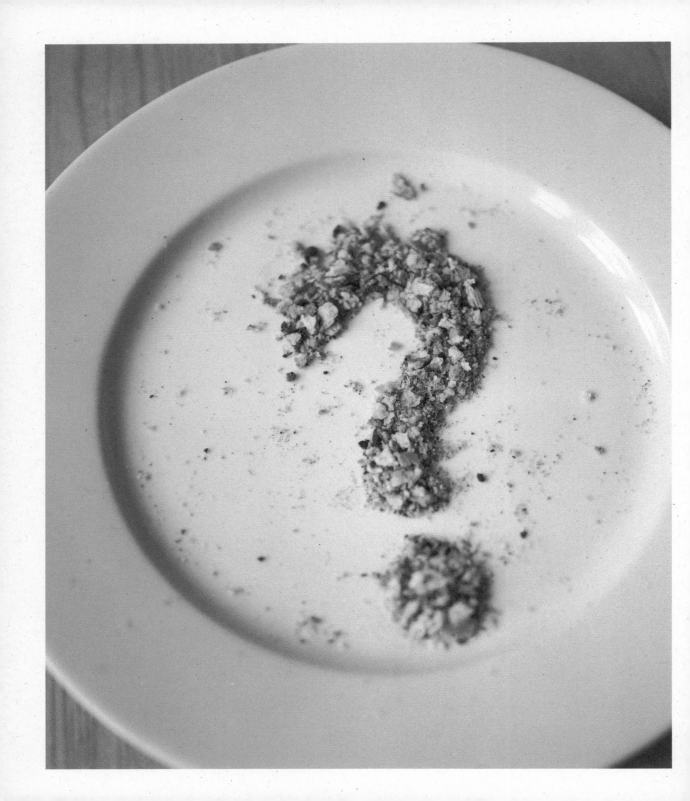

# Golden sandwich rules

Butter your bread right to the edges to prevent soggy sandwiches.

Wrap lunchbox sandwiches in greaseproof paper rather than clingfilm. No one likes a sweaty sandwich.

Always triangles. Never crust and bottom.

White bread releases sugars really quickly while wholegrain, rye and granary help you stay fuller for longer (and keep elasticated jeans at bay). Diehard white bread fan? Try half and half bread (page 284) as a compromise.

## Good places to eat your sandwiches
- The park bench
- The playground
- On a picnic blanket
- The beach (out of the wind in a secluded dune)

## Not so good places to eat your sandwiches
- Your desk
- Station platform
- The hairdresser's
- The beach (in the wind being pestered by wily seagulls)

## Sandwich sharing
- Ducks, pigeons and passing dogs = acceptable
- Traffic wardens, the monkeys down the zoo, strangers' children = less acceptable
- And swapping your fish-paste bap for someone else's cheese and chutney cobbler is just not sandwich cricket

# Pasta

The blank canvas of the pantry, the *tabula rasa* of teatime and the breakfast of everyone named Luigi, pasta is the culinary ocean on which 1000 sauces have been launched.

All these recipes take less than 10 minutes to make. Just enough time to get your pasta nice and al dente. They make enough sauce for around 150g of uncooked pasta. Just add an extra handful or so of the bigger ingredients if you're cooking for more.

Portion-wise, roughly 60g of pasta is about right for kids, while for grown-ups it's around 100g.

# Quick tomato sauce

**Ensure you always have a tin of tomatoes plus a few of the ingredients listed below knocking around and you'll never go hungry again.**

1 portion of your 5-a-day

olive oil

1 garlic clove, peeled and crushed

a handful of basil

1 x 400g tin of chopped tomatoes

Heat a good drizzle of olive oil in a pan and fry the garlic and basil over a high heat for about a minute. Add the chopped tomatoes, then turn down the heat and simmer for a couple of minutes, until the sauce has reduced.

Stir your cooked pasta into your sauce.

And if you like, throw a few of these staples into your pasta:

### Add any one of these
- A tin of tuna, drained
- A handful of cooked prawns
- 2 rashers of grilled bacon, chopped
- 4 slices of Parma ham, torn into strips
- 125g mozzarella cheese, torn into pieces

### Add as many of these as you like
- Olives
- Capers
- Roasted red pepper
- A handful of torn-up spinach or rocket
- Any leftover cooked vegetables
- Frozen peas

# THE SPOTTER'S GUIDE TO PASTA

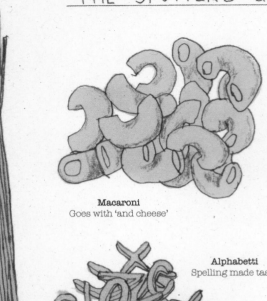

**Macaroni**
Goes with 'and cheese'

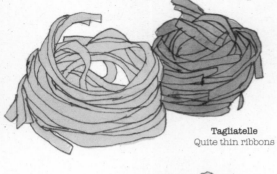

**Tagliatelle**
Quite thin ribbons

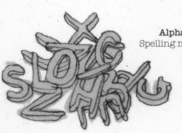

**Alphabetti**
Spelling made tasty

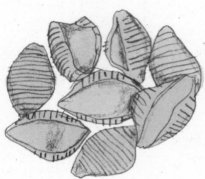

**Conchiglie**
She eats sea shells

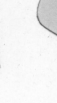

**Spaghetti**
Extremely thin ribbons

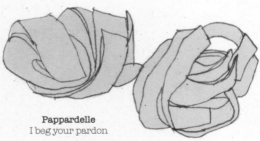

**Pappardelle**
I beg your pardon

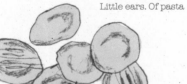

**Orecchiette**
Little ears. Of pasta

**Penne**
Not a fancy biro

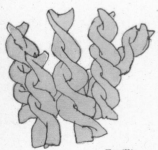

**Fusilli**
The twisty one

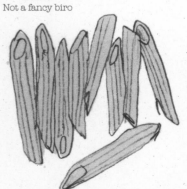

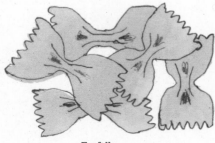

**Farfalle**
Action Man bowties

# THE SPOTTER'S GUIDE TO THINGS THAT GO WELL WITH PASTA

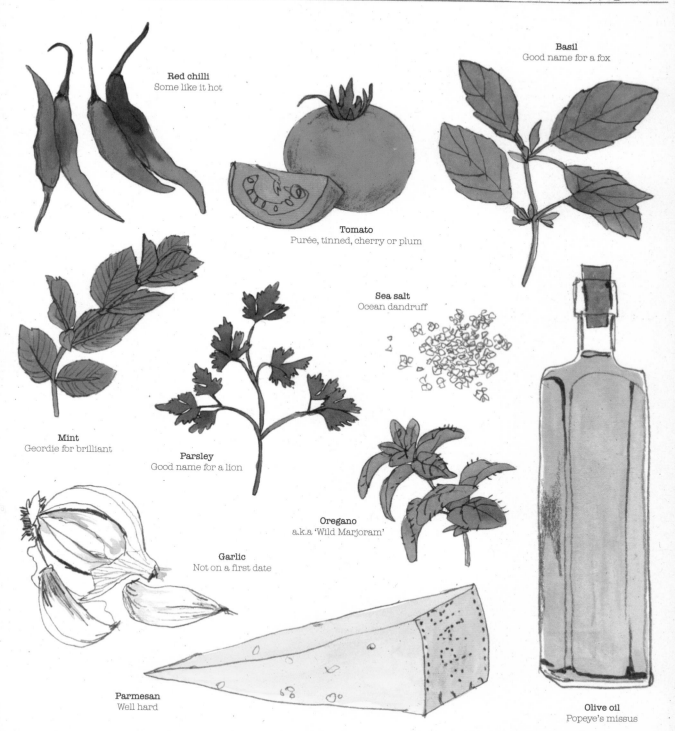

**Red chilli**
Some like it hot

**Tomato**
Purée, tinned, cherry or plum

**Basil**
Good name for a fox

**Mint**
Geordie for brilliant

**Parsley**
Good name for a lion

**Sea salt**
Ocean dandruff

**Oregano**
a.k.a 'Wild Marjoram'

**Garlic**
Not on a first date

**Parmesan**
Well hard

**Olive oil**
Popeye's missus

# Summer pasta

Both these recipes are light, fresh and perfect for dining al fresco. And they take minutes to prepare, meaning the kids won't get impatient and you get to make the most of the long summer days, without getting all cross over a hot stove first.

## Courgette and lemon

1 portion of your 5-a-day

2 courgettes, grated
zest and juice of 1 lemon
a couple of handfuls of freshly
  grated Parmesan cheese
a glug of olive oil
a handful of basil, chopped

Cook 150g linguine or spaghetti in a large pan of boiling water until al dente.

Meanwhile, grate the courgettes into a bowl and mix in the lemon zest and juice, the Parmesan, olive oil and basil.

Stir the courgette mixture straight into your hot drained pasta, along with a splash of the water it was cooked in. Season with salt and pepper and serve.

## Asparagus and spinach

1 portion of your 5-a-day

about 12 asparagus spears,
  a nice bunch
3 big handfuls of spinach
a handful of pine nuts
a handful of freshly grated
  Parmesan cheese

Cook 150g tagliatelle in a large pan of boiling water until al dente.

Chop the woody ends off the asparagus and discard. Whizz the spears in a food processor with the spinach, pine nuts and Parmesan.

Stir into the hot drained pasta, season with salt and pepper and serve.

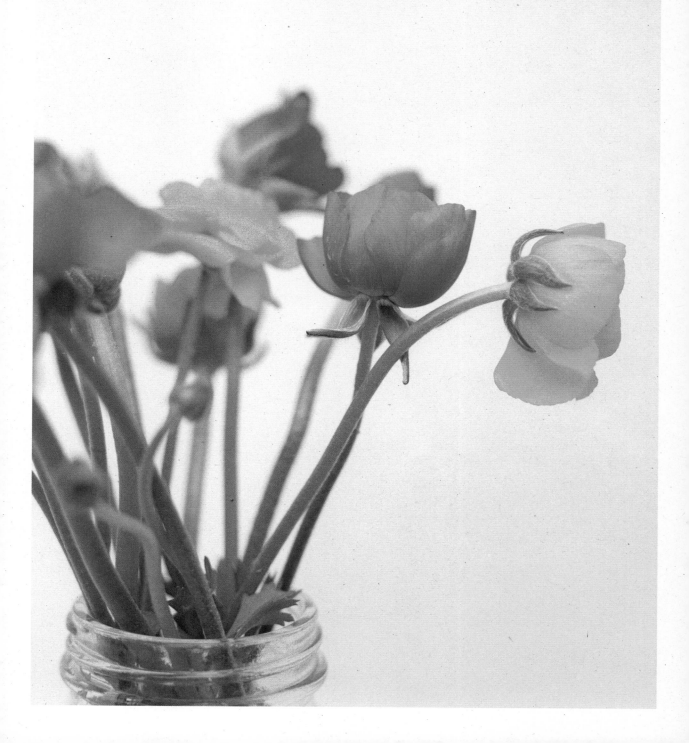

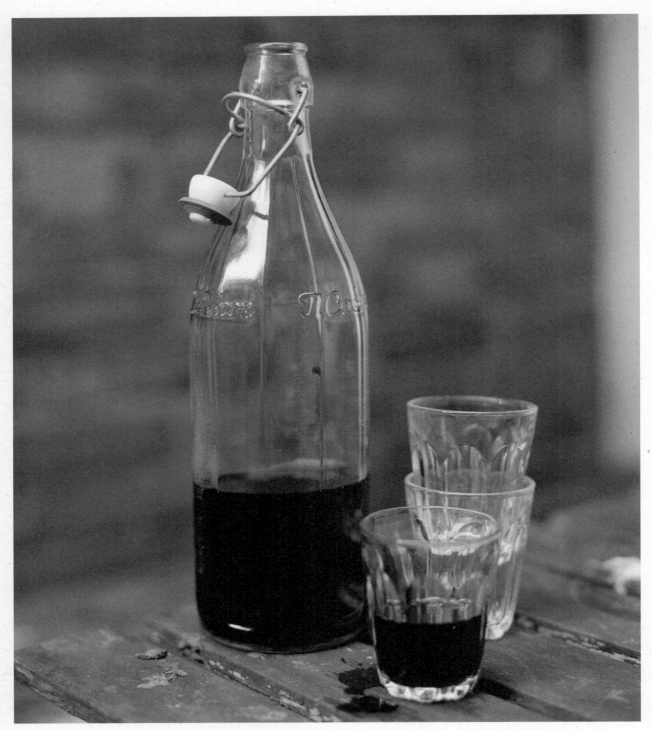

Red wine or Ribena – guess which this is.

# Winter pasta

Reclaim gloomy days by making one of these swift pasta dishes. For the right atmosphere, light a few candles and choose some appropriate music. There's one caveat – we guarantee the candles will get blown out pretty quickly (it's a weird condition kids have) so keep a torch handy.

## Quick carbonara

4 tablespoons crème fraîche
a couple of handfuls of freshly grated Parmesan cheese
4 rashers of bacon, grilled and chopped

Cook 150g penne in a large pan of boiling water until al dente.

Mix the crème fraîche and Parmesan in a bowl. Stir in the bacon.

Stir the crème fraîche mixture into the hot drained pasta with a splash of the water it was cooked in, and season well with salt and pepper.

## Red aubergines

1 portion of your 5-a-day

1 red pepper, roasted (or you can use a roasted red pepper from a jar)
olive oil
1 red onion, peeled and finely chopped
1 aubergine, cut into small chunks
1 x 400g tin of chopped tomatoes
a handful of chopped olives

Chop your roasted pepper. Cook 150g fusilli in a large pan of boiling salted water until al dente.

Heat a little olive oil in a pan and fry the onion until soft. Add the chopped pepper, aubergine and 3 tablespoons of water and simmer until the aubergine is soft. Add the tomatoes and olives and allow to simmer for another 10 minutes, until the sauce has reduced.

Stir into the hot drained pasta, season with salt and pepper, and serve with a sprinkling of freshly grated Parmesan.

Check out page 90 and 91 for pesto ideas.

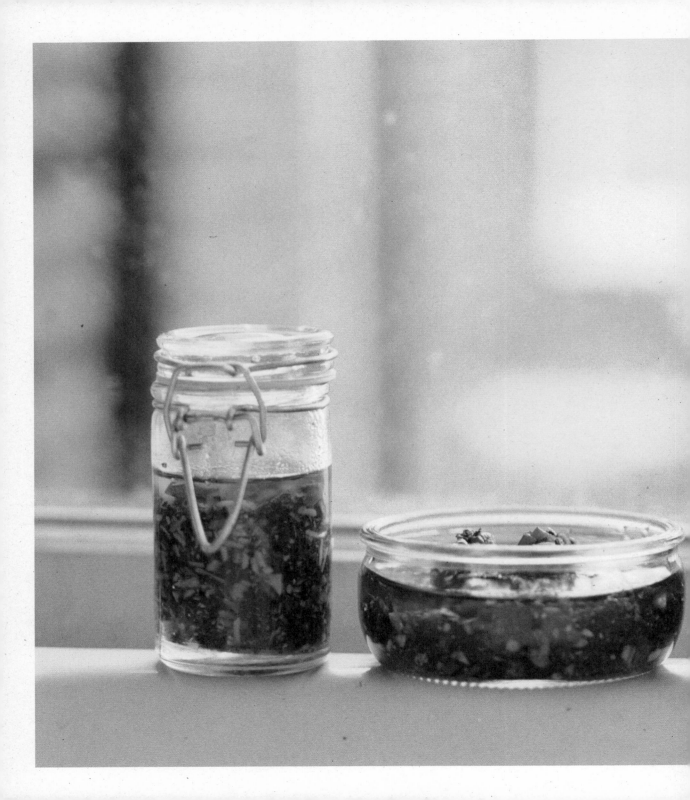

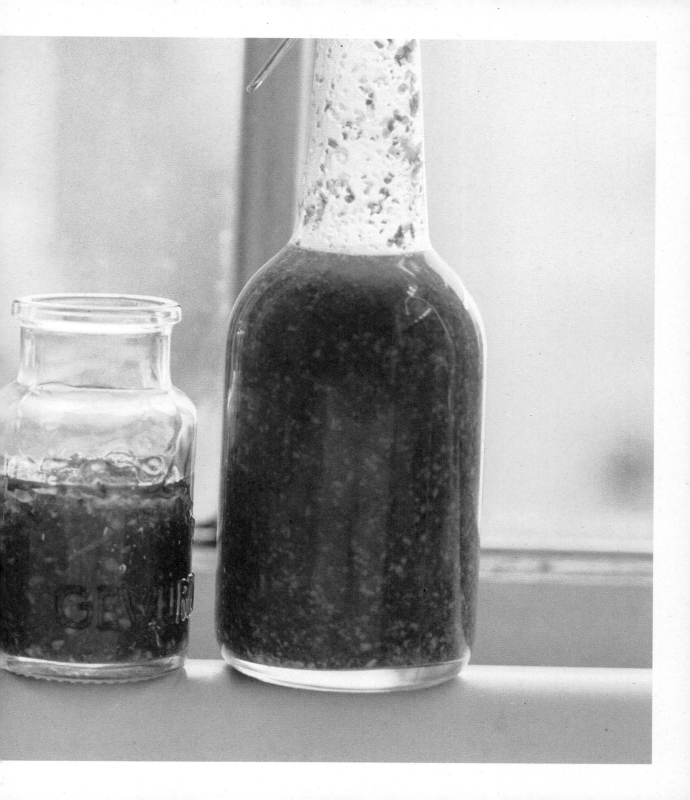

# MAKING PESTO
# IS REALLY EASY

Made in minutes, lasts for weeks (provided you keep it in the fridge), pesto is the answer to many a not-sure-what-to-make-for-tea dilemma. Just use the simple chart below as a guide and let indecisive meal times be a thing of the past. You can use a food processor or a pestle and mortar depending on how much time/bicep power you have.

|  | HERBS | NUTS | CHEESE | OIL | JUICE |
|---|---|---|---|---|---|
| SUMMER | 1 large bunch of basil | A small handful of pine nuts | A handful of grated Parmesan | A good glug of the best extra virgin olive oil you can get | The juice of 1 lemon |
| WINTER | 1 large bunch of parsley | A small handful of almonds | A handful of grated Manchego | A good glug of the best extra virgin olive oil you can get | The juice of 1 clementine |
| NOODLE | 1 large bunch of parsley | A small handful of cashews | A grated red chilli (not strictly a cheese, but does starts with ch) | A good glug of the best extra virgin olive oil you can get | The juice of 1 lime |
| MINTY | 1 large bunch of mint | A small handful of pistachios | A handful of grated pecorino | A good glug of the best extra virgin olive oil you can get | The juice of 1 lemon |

# HOW TO
# MAKE IT

First toast your nuts in a pan over a medium heat. Allow to cool and then make your pesto as below.

### Using a food processor?

Bung in half the citrus juice and all the other ingredients. Whizz until it looks like a pesto. Season with salt and pepper and have a taste. Add more juice if needed and more oil if it looks too thick.

### Using a pestle and mortar?

Bash the herbs with a pinch of sea salt into a thick green paste. Add the nuts and bash some more. Then add the cheese or chilli and grind into the paste.

Next add the oil and half the citrus juice and keep grinding until it looks like a pesto. Season with salt and pepper and taste. Add more juice if needed and more oil if it looks too thick.

# WHAT TO
# DO WITH IT

### GOOD STUFF TO DO WITH SUMMER PESTO

Stir through pasta or spread in toasted sandwiches. Spread over fish and roast in the oven at 200°C/400°F/gas mark 6 for 15 to 20 minutes.

Spread on a big slice of toasted ciabatta, top with 7 chopped cherry tomatoes and ½ a ball of mozzarella, torn into pieces for quick bruschetta.

### GOOD STUFF TO DO WITH WINTER PESTO

Spoon on top of stews and steaks. Spread in ham or cheese sandwiches. Stir into soup or dollop on to crispy roasted veg.

### GOOD STUFF TO DO WITH NOODLE PESTO

Spread over chicken breasts and roast in the oven at 200°C/400°F/ gas mark 6 for 20 minutes.

Use as a dressing for Asian veg, edamame beans or sugarsnap peas or just stir into a bowl of noodles.

### GOOD STUFF TO DO WITH MINTY PESTO

Stir through pasta with a handful of peas and some grated pecorino. Spoon on top of boiled new potatoes or mix into roasted courgettes as a side.

# SOUP GLORIOUS SOUP

The secret to all good soups is that they hail from the same humble beginnings. Just get the fractions right and, once you've mastered the basics, you can make all sorts of combinations.

### 1. THE BASE

2 cloves of garlic, peeled and finely chopped
1 carrot, peeled and chopped
1 medium onion, peeled and chopped
1 stick of celery, peeled and chopped
This is the foundation of your soup.

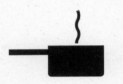

### 2. COOKED FLAVOURS

Woody herbs like rosemary and thyme, spices and cooked bacon all help to give your soup a richer flavour

### 3. THE HERO VEG

The main event of the soup

### 4. STOCK

Make sure you have enough chicken or vegetable stock to cover everything. If you don't have time to make your own, use good, organic, low salt stock cubes or bouillon

### 5. FINISHING TOUCHES

Just before serving, try adding some chopped herbs like mint and basil, a blob of fromage frais or plain yoghurt, or a sprinkling of toasted seeds

# HOW TO MAKE YOUR SOUP

The base stays the same for all soups.

Add the chopped base to a pan with a splash of olive oil and the cooked flavours. Cook on a medium for 10 to 15 minutes until soft.

Next add the chopped hero veg. The cooked base makes up about ⅕ of the soup, so your hero veg should make up the other ⅘.

Then add the stock to just cover everything and simmer until the veg is tender, tasting and seasoning as you go.

If you like your soups smooth, blitz with a hand blender. If you prefer them chunky, remove half, blitz the other half and then mix together.

Finally, add a finishing touch and serve up piping hot.
Turn over to pages 96 and 97 for some of our favourite soup suggestions.

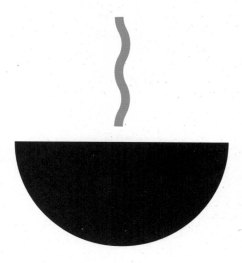

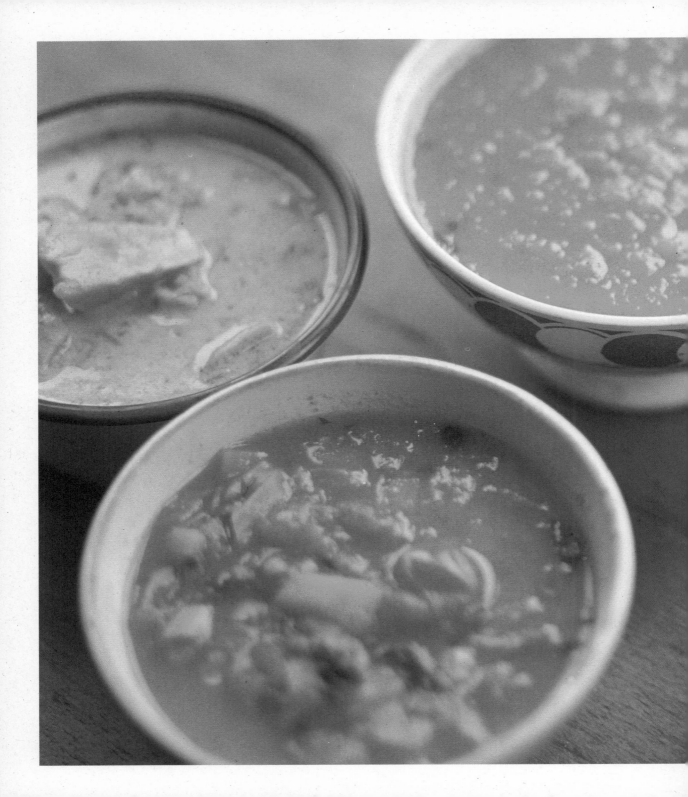

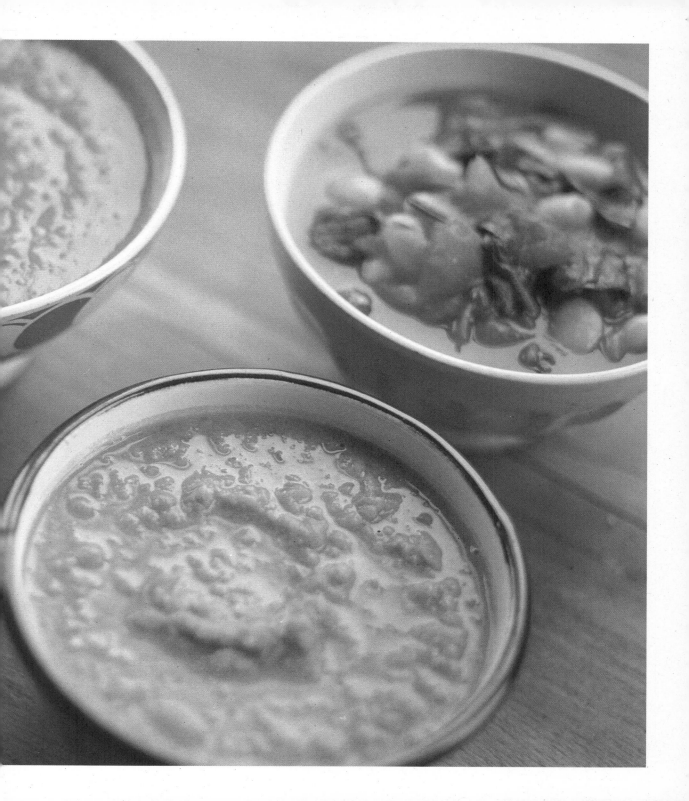

## Pea and bacon

Base – **see page 92**
Cooked – **3 rashers of bacon, chopped**
Hero veg – **6 handfuls of fresh/frozen peas**
Stock – **chicken or vegetable stock**
Finishing touches – **a dollop of fromage frais/plain yoghurt and some chopped mint**

## Butternut squash

Base – **see page 92**
Cooked – **a pinch of ground cinnamon, a pinch of dried chilli and the leaves from a sprig of rosemary**
Hero veg – **1 butternut squash, peeled and roughly chopped**
Stock – **chicken or vegetable stock**
Finishing touches – **a blob of fromage frais/plain yoghurt and some toasted pumpkin seeds**

## Tomato and basil

Base – **see page 92**
Cooked – **a small bunch of basil, roughly chopped**
Hero veg – **10 big ripe vine tomatoes**
Stock – **chicken or vegetable stock**
Finishing touches – **a dollop of fromage frais/plain yoghurt and more chopped basil**

## Spicy sweet potato

Base – **see page 92**
Cooked – **1 teaspoon of mustard seeds, 1 teaspoon of garam masala and 1 teaspoon of cumin seeds**
Hero veg – **4 medium sweet potatoes, peeled and roughly chopped**
Stock – **1 tin of coconut milk and chicken/vegetable stock to top up**
Finishing touches – **a blob of fromage frais/plain yoghurt and some fresh coriander**

## White bean and tomato

Base – see page 92
Cooked – leaves from 3 sprigs of rosemary
Hero veg – 4 large tomatoes, chopped, and a tin of cannellini or butter beans, drained and rinsed
Stock – vegetable stock
Finishing touches – stir in a few handfuls of fresh spinach and serve with a sprinkle of grated Parmesan cheese and a little drizzle of olive oil

## Your own soup recipe

**Jot down your favourite soup creation here:**

Base – see page 92
Cooked –
Hero veg –
Stock –
Finishing touches –


Bulk it up

- Chuck a handful of pasta, quinoa, or other grains into your soup 10 minutes before it's done.

- Or, if you have any leftover soup, you can add cooked pasta or grains afterwards.

- Tinned lentils and beans are a great way to add protein to your soup as well as bulking it up a bit.

All these soups freeze well, so make up double batches and freeze in old takeaway containers for a satisfying freezer-full of meals you can make in minutes.

# GOOD THINGS TO HAVE FOR

---

# SNACKS

# Honey and cinnamon popcorn

This recipe is for honey and cinnamon popcorn but you can use maple syrup or salty butter or even a mixture of the two. No holds barred in crazy old Corn Town. Bag it up for a trip to the pictures or pile high into your biggest bowl and settle down to watch *Dumbo*.

Makes loads

a splash of vegetable, sunflower or groundnut oil
2 handfuls of popcorn kernels
4 tablespoons runny honey
a pinch of ground cinnamon

Find a big pan with a lid. Add a tiny splash of oil and the popcorn kernels. Put the lid on and cook over a very low heat. At first you won't hear a thing, but once the popping starts, keep giving the pan a gentle shake every minute or so until the noise stops. Then turn off the heat.

In another pan, heat the honey and cinnamon over a low heat for a couple of minutes.

Put the popcorn on to a large baking tray and pour over the honey mixture. Give the tray a good shake and stir the popcorn with a spoon to make sure it's well coated. Pop the tray back into the oven for 3 to 5 minutes, to set the honey, then remove and leave to cool.

Once cooled, either serve in little bowls straight away or keep in an airtight tin for up to a week, and have some sandwich bags ready for when you next pop out (sorry).

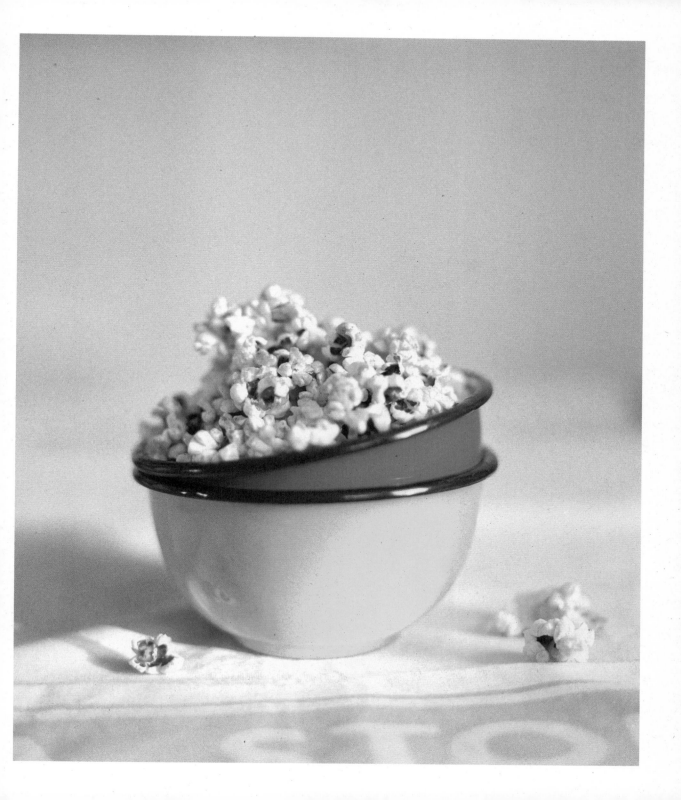

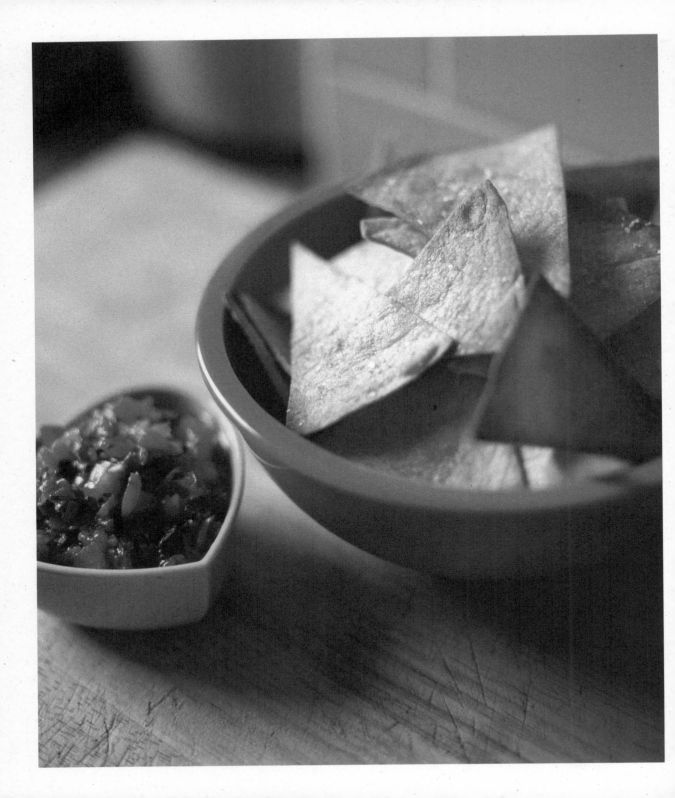

# Homemade tortilla chips and salsa dip

Think of these tortilla chips as mini, crispy boats, ready to transport a cargo of rich tomato salsa to hungry mouths everywhere. Enough to see you through an entire episode of *Doctor Who*. All aboard the good ship, er, Chip.

Makes enough for one decent film/movie

counts towards your 5-a-day

For the chips

8 flour tortillas, wraps or pitta breads
olive oil
1 teaspoon smoked paprika
salt, if needed

For the salsa dip

4 ripe tomatoes
2 spring onions
a small bunch of coriander
½ a red chilli, deseeded
juice of ½ a lime
extra virgin olive oil

Preheat your oven to 180°C/350°F/gas mark 4.

Cut each tortilla into 8 triangles and place them on a couple of baking trays.

Drizzle with olive oil, sprinkle with smoked paprika and toss the chips to make sure they're all coated. Add a pinch of salt if you like.

Bake for 10 minutes, until crispy, then remove from the oven.

Next, make your salsa. Roughly chop the tomatoes, spring onions, coriander and chilli on a big board. Then, using a large knife, sweep and chop them all together until well diced. Place in a bowl.

Squeeze over the lime juice, drizzle with olive oil, season and mix together. Taste to see if the flavours are balanced, and add a bit more lime, oil or salt if you think it's needed.

Alternatively, if you're really short of time, you can bung the whole lot into a food processor and whizz until chunky.

Then check the seasoning and serve with the tortilla chips.

# How to make their popcorn last for an entire DVD

You've got a bowl of popcorn. You've sat down with your kids and they've picked the film. Two things are certain. One, you will inevitably end up quite enjoying their film. Two, they will eat all the popcorn before the studio logos at the start have finished. So here's a quick guide to enjoying some of our tried and tested favourites whilst making the kids ration the homemade snacks.

Eat 3 bits of popcorn every time Marge gets cross with Homer

Eat 3 bits of popcorn any time a grown up is mean

Eat 4 bits of popcorn whenever somebody goes underwater

Eat 8 bits of popcorn when you see a boy in a vest

Eat 3 bits of popcorn for every tiara or shiny dress you can spot

Eat 1 bit of popcorn every time you hear 'Yo' or 'Ho'

Eat 3 bits of popcorn whenever you see a pheasant

Eat 3 bits of popcorn every time a new monster appears

Eat 7 bits of popcorn every time you see maple syrup

Eat 4 bits of popcorn whenever you see Oscar the Grouch

Eat 10 bits of popcorn every time Spidey's senses tingle

Eat 10 bits of popcorn every time you feel a bit teary

Eat 3 bits of popcorn for every animal that breaks into song

Eat one twentieth of a bit of popcorn when you see a fish

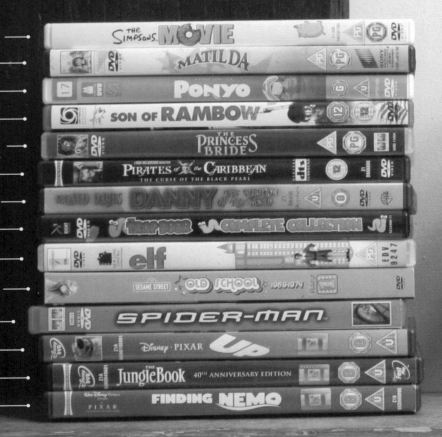

# How to make your tortillas last for an entire night in

The kids are in bed. Or at a friend's house. Or anywhere really, but most importantly, they're not in front of the TV. Your TV. You've made tortillas specially but the excitement of holding the remote is making you want to devour them. Don't. Spread them out during some of our favourites with this handy guide.

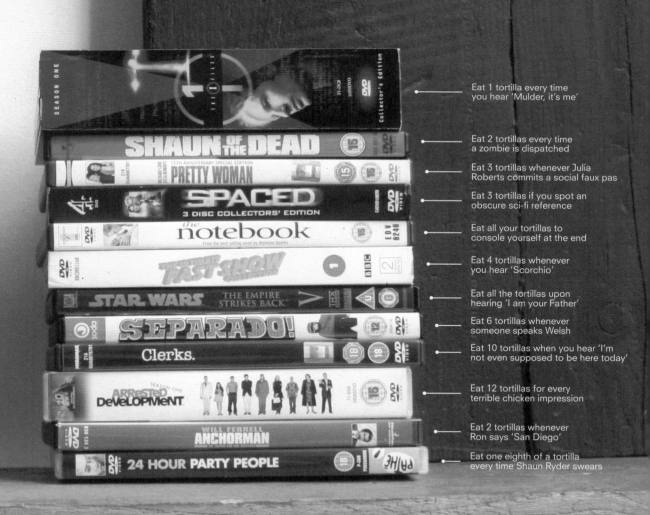

Eat 1 tortilla every time you hear 'Mulder, it's me'

Eat 2 tortillas every time a zombie is dispatched

Eat 3 tortillas whenever Julia Roberts commits a social faux pas

Eat 3 tortillas if you spot an obscure sci-fi reference

Eat all your tortillas to console yourself at the end

Eat 4 tortillas whenever you hear 'Scorchio'

Eat all the tortillas upon hearing 'I am your Father'

Eat 6 tortillas whenever someone speaks Welsh

Eat 10 tortillas when you hear 'I'm not even supposed to be here today'

Eat 12 tortillas for every terrible chicken impression

Eat 2 tortillas whenever Ron says 'San Diego'

Eat one eighth of a tortilla every time Shaun Ryder swears

# Some good dips

Dips are a clever way to get loads of veg into anyone. These all count towards your 5-a-day. Bingo.

### Yellow hummus

Fry the cumin seeds in a dry frying pan for a minute or two until lightly toasted and smelling good. Then bash them in the pestle and mortar.

Put the ground-up cumin seeds into a bowl with the chickpeas, tahini, olive oil, lemon zest and juice, and use a hand blender to whizz to a paste. If you have a food processor, just pulse everything in there.

### Green hummus

Put the courgettes, tahini, olive oil, lemon zest and juice into a bowl and use a hand blender to whizz to a smooth paste. Add the mint right at the end and give it another whizz. Or, if you have a food processor, just chuck everything in there and pulse away.

### Red hummus

Dry fry the coriander seeds for a minute or two until they begin to release their aromas. Then give them a good grinding in the pestle and mortar. Put the coriander seeds, beetroots, tahini, olive oil, clementine zest and juice into a bowl and use a hand blender to whizz to a paste or blend the whole lot in a food processor.

### Pea-green dip

Put the peas into a deep bowl and cover with boiling water. Leave for 3 minutes, then drain them and return them to the bowl. Add the rest of the ingredients, then use a hand blender to whizz until smooth. Or pop everything into a food processor and pulse away.

Try stirring into pasta with a little grated Parmesan or spoon on to a baked potato with some rocket for a quick tasty lunch.

Makes a good bowlful
1 teaspoon cumin seeds, crushed
1 x 400g tin of chickpeas, drained and rinsed
1 teaspoon tahini
1 tablespoon olive oil
zest and juice of 1 lemon

Makes a decent bowlful
2 big courgettes, roughly chopped
1 teaspoon tahini
1 tablespoon olive oil
zest and juice of 1 lemon
a handful of fresh mint

Makes a hearty bowlful
1 teaspoon coriander seeds
4 cooked beetroots
1 teaspoon tahini
1 tablespoon olive oil
zest and juice of 1 clementine

Serves 2 for lunch, or
4 for snacking

6 big handfuls of frozen peas
a bunch of mint
3 tablespoons plain yoghurt
zest and juice of 1 lemon

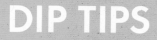

# DIP TIPS

## GOOD THINGS FOR DIPPING

Carrots, radishes, cucumber, baby courgettes,
chicory leaves, little gem leaves and celery.

## PROPER DIPPING ETIQUETTE

If your crisp breaks off, don't go back for it.

Fingers are not dipping implements. Even when all the carrot sticks are finished.

Dainty dipping makes for longer lasting dips and is a sure-fire way to get invited back round for tea.

Scooping the entire lot on to a single tortilla chip will guarantee the opposite.

Never ever ever double dip.

## STORING YOUR DIPS

Your dips will keep in a big tub in the fridge for up to 7 days. Try:

Popping into little pots for lunches or outings, with some vegetables for dipping.

Spreading on sandwiches as another way to get a portion of veg ticked off.

Serving as a healthy after-school snack with homemade tortilla chips (page 103),
cheese twigs (page 286), oatcakes, rice cakes or crispbreads.

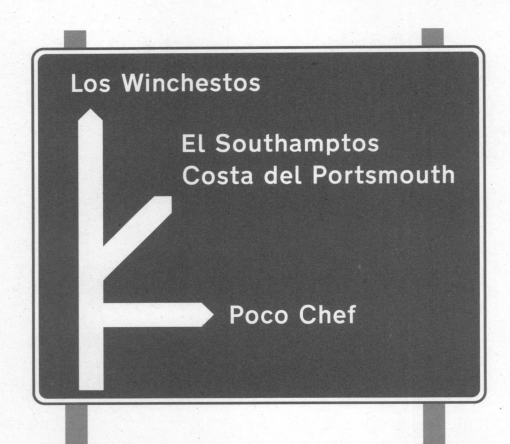

# Quesadillas

**Brilliant vehicles for leftovers, quick snacks and party food. Less brilliant for driving down the A34 to Winchester.**

Serves 4
1 portion of your 5-a-day

For the quesadillas
4 flour tortillas
150g Cheddar cheese, grated
1 carrot or courgette, grated
1 red chilli, deseeded and
   finely chopped
1 spring onion, finely chopped

For the dip
1 avocado
7 cherry tomatoes, diced
juice of 1 lime

Lay out the tortillas on a clean flat surface.

Put the cheese, carrot or courgette, chilli and spring onion into a bowl and mix well.

Divide the mixture in half and spread over 2 of the tortilla wraps. Lay the other 2 wraps on top and press down to stick them together.

Cut the avocado in half and remove the stone, then mash the flesh in a bowl with the cherry tomatoes and lime juice. Season well with salt and pepper.

Heat a frying pan big enough to fit one of your quesadillas (these are best made in a dry pan). Carefully place one of the quesadillas in the pan and toast for 2 to 3 minutes, until golden underneath.

Use a fish slice to flip over and cook on the other side for a further 2 minutes. By now the cheese should have melted and stuck the tortillas together.

Remove from the heat to a chopping board and cook the other quesadilla the same way.

Cut the quesadillas into wedges and serve with the avocado dip. Or try them with one of the salads on pages 211 to 223 for a slightly heartier lunch.

# WHAT'S FOR DINNER?

Not sure what to have for tea tonight? Let the Dinner Decider™ choose your plate's fate. Get an A4 piece of paper, follow the folding instructions below and may your next meal never be more than a quick flick-pick-and-a-nip-down-the-shops away.

▼ ▼ ▼ ▼ ▼ ▼ ▼ ▼ ▼ ▼

### 1

Turn your paper this way round and fold the bottom right-hand corner to the left-hand edge

### 2

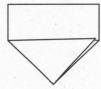

Then fold the bottom left-hand corner to the right-hand edge

### 3

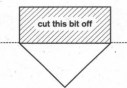

cut this bit off

Next, cut off the rectangle bit and put to one side to write your shopping list on later

### 4

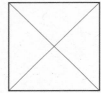

Then open out your paper and lay it out in front of you

### 5

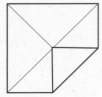

Fold each corner into the centre

### 6

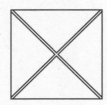

Your paper should end up looking like the back of a big square envelope

### 7

Once you've folded all the corners in, turn your paper over...

### 8

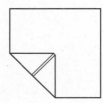

...and fold each corner back on itself into the centre

**9**

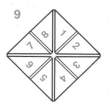

Then write the
numbers 1–8 on each
little triangle

**10**

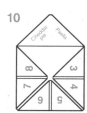

Under each flap write
a selection of recipes
from the dinner section
(p.112-193). Two per flap

**11**

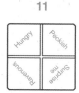

Next, fold the flaps back
down and then turn over
to the blank side. On each
square, write down how
hungry you are

**12**

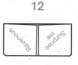

Fold in half so that the
edges line up and
repeat on the other
side so that creases
are nice and sharp

**14**

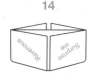

Turn your decider upside
down and push your index
fingers into the top two
corners and your thumbs
into the bottom two corners

**15**

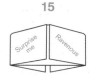

Then pinch together so
your decider folds up
into a funny star shape

**16**

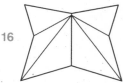

Have a few practice
flicks before picking
your dinner

### How to use your finished Dinner Decider™

1. To decide what's on the menu tonight, choose one of the words in the
squares and spell it out using one flick per letter (e.g. Hungry = 6 flicks).

2. Next choose a number and count it out, flick by flick.

3. Then choose another number, lift up the flap and voilà – that's what
you're having for tea tonight. If we lost you round about step 4, just ask
any girl over the age of 12 to show you the ropes. We guarantee they'll
know what to do, they're born with the knowledge.

TM = Tasty Meals

GOOD THINGS TO HAVE FOR DINNER

---

# VEGGIE

# 5 reasons to eat in season

**It's good for you**

Trying new things, getting a mixture of nutrients, inventing clever ways to jazz up a cabbage. Much more fun than same old, same old.

**It's good for the planet**

Less air-freighted Kenyan French beans = less carbon emissions, less pollution, less environmental impact, better chance of not kippering the planet.

**It's more natural**

Forcing stuff to grow when it's not meant to is just plain weird (apart from rhubarb). Mother Nature created seasons for a reason. And she knows her stuff.

**It's cheaper**

You try getting change from a fiver if you nip out to buy a bag of cherries in March.

**The best things come to those who wait**

There's a certain satisfaction that comes with having to wait a bit. The excitement at tasting the first strawberry of summer. The countdown to roasted Brussels sprouts. It's all about delayed gratification.

|  |  |
|---|---|
| **January** | Apples, **beetroots**, Brussels sprouts, **cabbage,** |
| **February** | Apples, **beetroots**, Brussels sprouts, **cabbage,** |
| **March** | Apples, **beetroots**, Brussels sprouts, **cabbage,** celery, |
| **April** | Apples, **cabbage,** celeriac, **kale,** leeks, **parsnips,** |
| **May** | **Asparagus,** broad beans, **cabbage,** gooseberries, |
| **June** | **Asparagus,** broad beans, **broccoli,** cabbage, **celery,** |
| **July** | **Apricots,** broad beans, **beetroots,** broccoli, rhubarb, **runner beans,** strawberries, **tomatoes,** |
| **August** | Apples, **apricots,** beetroots, **broccoli,** peas, **peaches,** peppers, radishes, **raspberries,** |
| **September** | Apples, **apricots,** beetroots, **Brussels sprouts,** **peaches,** pears, **peppers,** plums, **pumpkin,** |
| **October** | Apples, **Brussels sprouts,** blackberries, **cabbage,** red cabbage, **swede,** sweetcorn, **tomatoes,** turnips. |
| **November** | Apples, **beetroots,** Brussels sprouts, **cabbage,** **red cabbage,** swede, **turnips.** |
| **December** | **Brussels sprouts,** cabbage, **cauliflower,** celery, |

cauliflower, **celeriac**, celery, **cooking apples**, kale, **leeks**, parsnips, **swede**, turnips.

cauliflower, **celeriac**, celery, **cooking apples**, kale, **leeks**, purple sprouting broccoli, **red cabbage**, rhubarb, **swede**, turnips.

kale, **leeks**, parsnips, **purple sprouting broccoli**, radishes, **red cabbage**, rhubarb, **spring greens**, swede.

pears, **purple sprouting broccoli**, radishes, **rhubarb**, spring greens, **watercress**.

**new potatoes**, parsnips, **purple sprouting broccoli**, radishes, **rhubarb**, spring greens, **watercress**.

cherries, **courgettes**, French beans, **new potatoes**, peas, **radishes**, rhubarb, **runner beans**, strawberries, **tomatoes**, watercress.

**blackcurrants**, cabbage, **cherries**, courgettes, **French beans**, new potatoes, **peas**, peaches, **peppers**, radishes, **raspberries**, watercress.

blackcurrants, **beans (runner and French)**, cabbage, **cauliflower**, celery, **cherries**, courgettes, **gooseberries**, leeks, **marrows**, strawberries, **sweetcorn**, tomatoes, **watercress**.

blackberries, **cabbage**, cauliflower, **celery**, courgettes, **field mushrooms**, gooseberries, **leeks**, marrows, **parsnips**, peas, radishes, **raspberries**, swede, **sweetcorn**.

cauliflower, **celery**, courgettes, **chestnuts**, cooking apples, **cranberries**, field mushrooms, **kale**, leeks, **parsnips**, **pumpkins**,

cauliflower, **celery**, chestnuts, **cooking apples**, cranberries, **field mushrooms**, kale, **leeks**, parsnips, **pears**, pumpkins,

**chestnuts**, cranberries, **field mushrooms**, kale, **leeks**, parsnips, red cabbage, **swede**, turnips.

**THINGS THAT ARE AVAILABLE ALL YEAR ROUND:**
Onions, carrots, chard, mushrooms, spinach, garlic, potatoes, salad leaves, baked beans.

# Veggie burgers

**There are six different vegetables hidden in between the baps of these burgers. They need about 20 minutes in the fridge before cooking so why not make a double batch, wrap half in clingfilm and freeze for another time and thank yourself in advance.**

Put all the potatoes into a pan of boiling water and bring back to the boil. Chuck in the peas, bring back to the boil again, and simmer for 5 minutes. Scoop out the potatoes with a slotted spoon, then drain the peas. Leaving the spuds to one side to cool, return the peas to the pan and mash with a potato masher.

Heat a little olive oil in a frying pan and cook the spring onions and spices for a minute or two, until soft. Turn off the heat.

Put the grated carrot, courgette, halloumi and chopped mint into a big bowl and grate in the cooled potatoes. Mix well. Add the peas, spring onions, egg, flour and breadcrumbs to the bowl and season as needed (don't forget that the halloumi is already quite salty).

Wet your hands to stop the mixture sticking to them, and give the whole lot a really good mix. Then divide the mixture into 4, and mould and shape each portion into a round pattie. Pop the patties into the fridge for at least 20 minutes, or as long as you've got, to let them firm up a bit. Meanwhile, preheat your oven to 200°C/400°F/gas mark 6.

When the patties have had their time in the fridge, put them on a baking tray, drizzle them with olive oil and bake in the oven for 25 to 30 minutes, until golden brown.

Toast your bread rolls and serve the burgers sandwiched between them, layered with sliced tomato, lettuce leaves, a good dollop of homemade traffic-light ketchup (page 310), some rainbow chips (page 224) and chop chop salad (page 220).

Makes 4 burgers
(or 8 kid-sized ones)
2 portions of your 5-a-day

For the burgers

1 sweet potato, peeled and
    cut into big chunks
2 large waxy potatoes,
    peeled and cut into small
    chunks
a small handful of frozen peas
olive oil
4 spring onions, finely
    chopped
1 teaspoon smoked paprika
1 teaspoon ground cumin
1 carrot, peeled and grated
1 courgette, grated
100g halloumi cheese, grated
a couple of sprigs of mint
1 large free-range egg
2 tablespoons plain flour
a big handful of brown
    breadcrumbs

For the topping

4 of your favourite bread rolls
3 big tomatoes, sliced
a big handful of lettuce leaves

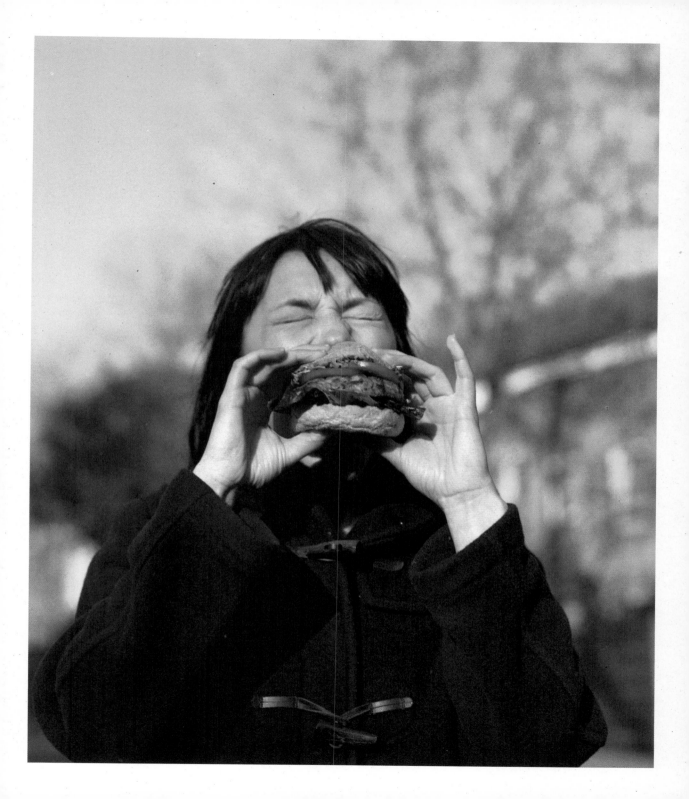

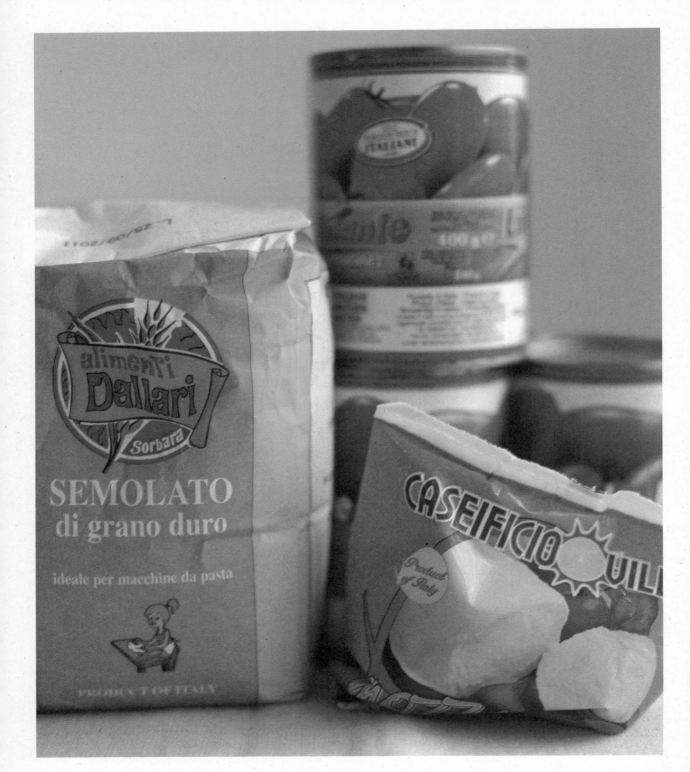

# Gnocchi alla Romana

Eaten by the Romans when they went for a stomp, these little dumplings are easy to make and work well with just about any pasta sauce you care to throw at them. Yet another thing (along with straight roads, central heating and novelty calendars) to thank them for.

Serves 4 (makes about 40 gnocchi, depending on size)
1 portion of your 5-a-day

For the gnocchi
200ml milk
125g coarse semolina
2 free-range egg yolks
a good grating of nutmeg
15g butter
125g mozzarella (roughly one big ball)
50g Parmesan cheese, freshly grated

For the tomato sauce
olive oil
1 onion, peeled and finely chopped
1 garlic clove, peeled and finely chopped
1 small carrot, peeled and finely chopped
a sprig of thyme
a sprig of rosemary
1 x 400g tin of chopped plum tomatoes

Put the milk into a saucepan with 150ml water and a pinch of salt and bring to the boil. Turn down the heat and slowly pour in the semolina, using a whisk to stir constantly until the mixture has come together. This will take about 10 minutes.

Turn off the heat and leave to cool for 10 minutes or so, then stir in the egg yolks, nutmeg, butter and a pinch of salt and pepper.

Using a spatula, spread the mixture about 1cm thick on a well-oiled baking tray and leave to cool completely.

Heat a splash of olive oil in a second pan for the tomato sauce and cook the onion, garlic, carrot and herbs over a low heat for 5 to 10 minutes, until soft. Stir in the tomatoes and season with salt and pepper. Put a lid on the pan and leave to simmer for about 15 minutes, adding a little water if needed.

Preheat your oven to 180°C/350°F/gas mark 4.

Once your gnocchi mix is cold, use a round pastry cutter or a glass to cut out little circles (about 4-5cm in diameter). Arrange them in a buttered baking dish so that they are slightly overlapping one another.

Break up the mozzarella and dot it over the top of the gnocchi, then sprinkle with the grated Parmesan and bake in the oven for 10 minutes.

Serve the gnocchi (about 10 per person) with the rich tomato sauce poured over, and with a big green salad (page 211) and a hunk of tomato and thyme focaccia (page 282) or granary bread.

# Oven-baked squash risotto

According to grain pedants, in order to be officially called a risotto, the rice must be fried in butter, doused in wine, simmered in stock, constantly stirred and eaten off a flat dish. However, the rice police will not be informed if you go off-piste with this recipe. Especially if you don't answer the door to them.

1 portion of your 5-a-day

1 butternut squash, peeled and cut into small chunks
1 red chilli, deseeded and roughly chopped
a few sprigs of rosemary
olive oil
1 onion, peeled and finely chopped
1 stick of celery, finely chopped
300g risotto rice
a small glass of white wine
1 litre hot vegetable stock
a knob of butter
a sprinkling of freshly grated Parmesan cheese

Preheat the oven to 180°C/350°F/gas mark 4.

Put the squash, chilli and rosemary into a sturdy deep-sided roasting tray. Drizzle with olive oil, season with salt and pepper and give the tin a good shake. Roast in the oven for 30 to 40 minutes, until the squash is golden.

Meanwhile, heat a drizzle of oil in a large pan and cook the onion and celery for 10 to 15 minutes, until soft and translucent. Add the rice and cook for a few minutes, then pour in the wine and allow to reduce down.

Take the squash out of the oven, remove the rosemary sprigs, and gently mash, then add the rice mixture and pour over the hot stock. Give it a stir, then put back into the oven and bake for another 20 to 30 minutes, or until all the liquid has been absorbed.

Finally, stir in the butter and grated Parmesan and serve with a simple rocket salad and a few shavings of fresh Parmesan.

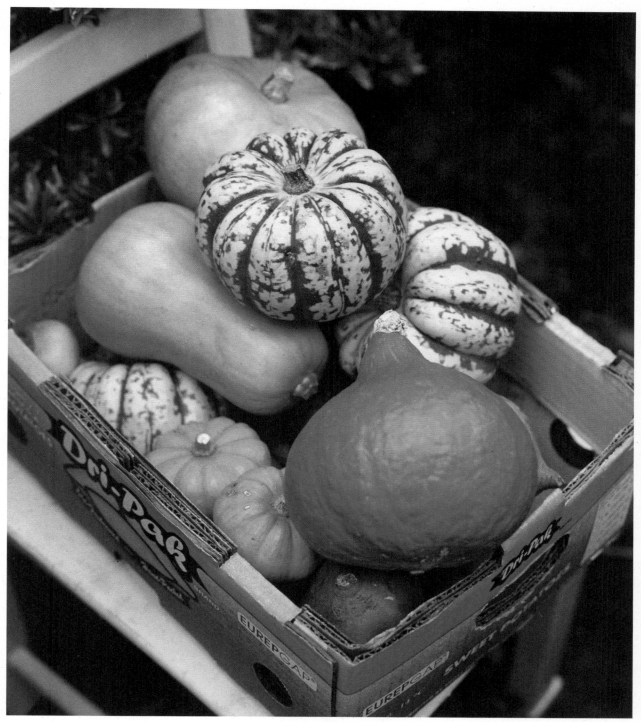

Looks like a bit of a squash (you're fired, *Ed*).

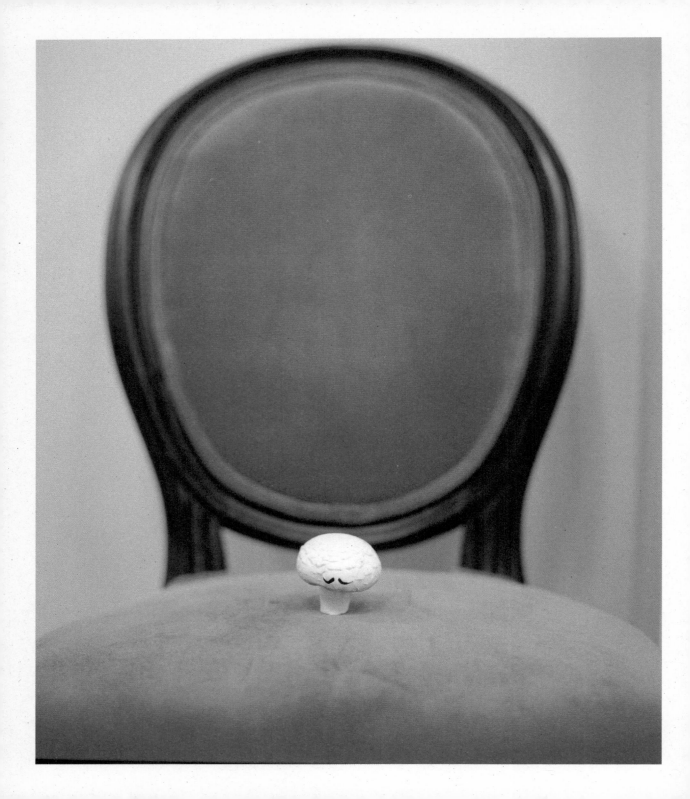

# Posh mushroom pasta bake

According to mushroom enthusiasts, the world's poshest mushroom is the Japanese matsutake mushroom. Given that these fun guys cost around $200 a pop, we plumped for cooking the bog-standard variety in a fancy (yet more purse-friendly) manner. For those expecting a more aristocratic affair, please accept this photo of a rather splendid chap as compensation.

**Serves 4**

1½ portions of your 5-a-day

a small handful of dried porcini

400g mushrooms, a mix of wild and cultivated flat ones

olive oil

2 big leeks, washed, trimmed and finely chopped

4 garlic cloves, peeled and finely sliced

1 small bunch of thyme, stalks removed

a glass of white wine

350g spaghetti

150ml single cream

100g fresh spinach

zest of 1 lemon

150g freshly grated Parmesan cheese

Preheat your oven to 180°C/350°F/gas mark 4.

Put the porcini into a bowl and cover them with 150ml boiling water. If you're using wild mushrooms, clean them well. Then slice or tear the flat ones and leave to one side.

Heat a drizzle of olive oil in a large frying pan and cook the leeks, garlic and thyme for about 10 minutes, until soft.

Add the mushrooms and cook until browned. Then add the porcini with their liquid and the wine. Allow to bubble for 10 minutes, until the sauce has reduced down. While you're waiting for the sauce to reduce, cook the spaghetti in a big pan of salted boiling water for a couple of minutes fewer than it says on the packet. Drain, return to the pan and leave to one side.

Pour the cream into your sauce, bring to the boil and then turn off the heat. Stir the sauce and spinach into the cooked pasta along with the lemon zest and about two-thirds of the Parmesan.

Then tip the lot into a big oven dish, sprinkle with the remaining Parmesan and bake for 35 to 40 minutes, till golden and crispy.

Serve with a big green salad (page 211).

# Green mac and cheese

Tucked away under a crunchy, green canopy of blitzed-up broccoli, tiny jewels of roasted butternut squash happily nestle amidst creamy macaroni. If you're lucky, you might even see the Lesser Spotted Cherry Tomato. All depends on how you spoon it on to the plate.

Serves 4
1 portion of your 5-a-day

½ a butternut squash, peeled, deseeded and cut into little chunks
olive oil
a big bunch of basil, stalks removed
2 slices of good-quality brown bread, stale or dried out in the oven
½ a small head of broccoli (about 100g), roughly chopped
4 tablespoons crème fraîche
100g Cheddar cheese, grated
100g Manchego cheese, grated
a large handful of cherry tomatoes
300g macaroni

Preheat your oven to 200°C/400°F/gas mark 6 and put a large pan of water on to boil.

Put the squash pieces in a roasting tray. Drizzle with oil, add a pinch of salt and pepper and roast for about 25 minutes, till golden.

Put half the basil, all the bread, the broccoli and a good splash of olive oil into a food processor and whizz to fine breadcrumbs. Transfer to a bowl and set aside. Give the food processor a clean.

Mix the crème fraîche and grated cheeses together in a bowl. Put the cherry tomatoes and the rest of the basil into the food processor, pulse a couple of times, then tip into the crème fraîche mixture.

When the squash has about 10 minutes of roasting time left to go, chuck the pasta into the pan of boiling water and cook for a couple of minutes fewer than the packet says – you want it slightly undercooked.

Once the pasta and squash are ready, scoop out a mugful of the pasta water and set aside.

Drain the pasta in a colander, then pop it back into the pan and pour over the cheesy mixture. Add the roasted squash and give it all a good stir, using the pasta water to help give the sauce the consistency of single cream. The pasta will soak up the sauce once you bake it, so it needs to go into the oven a little runny.

Pour the whole lot into a baking dish, spread the green breadcrumbs evenly over the top and bake in the oven for 25 minutes, until the breadcrumbs are crunchy. Serve with chop chop salad (page 220).

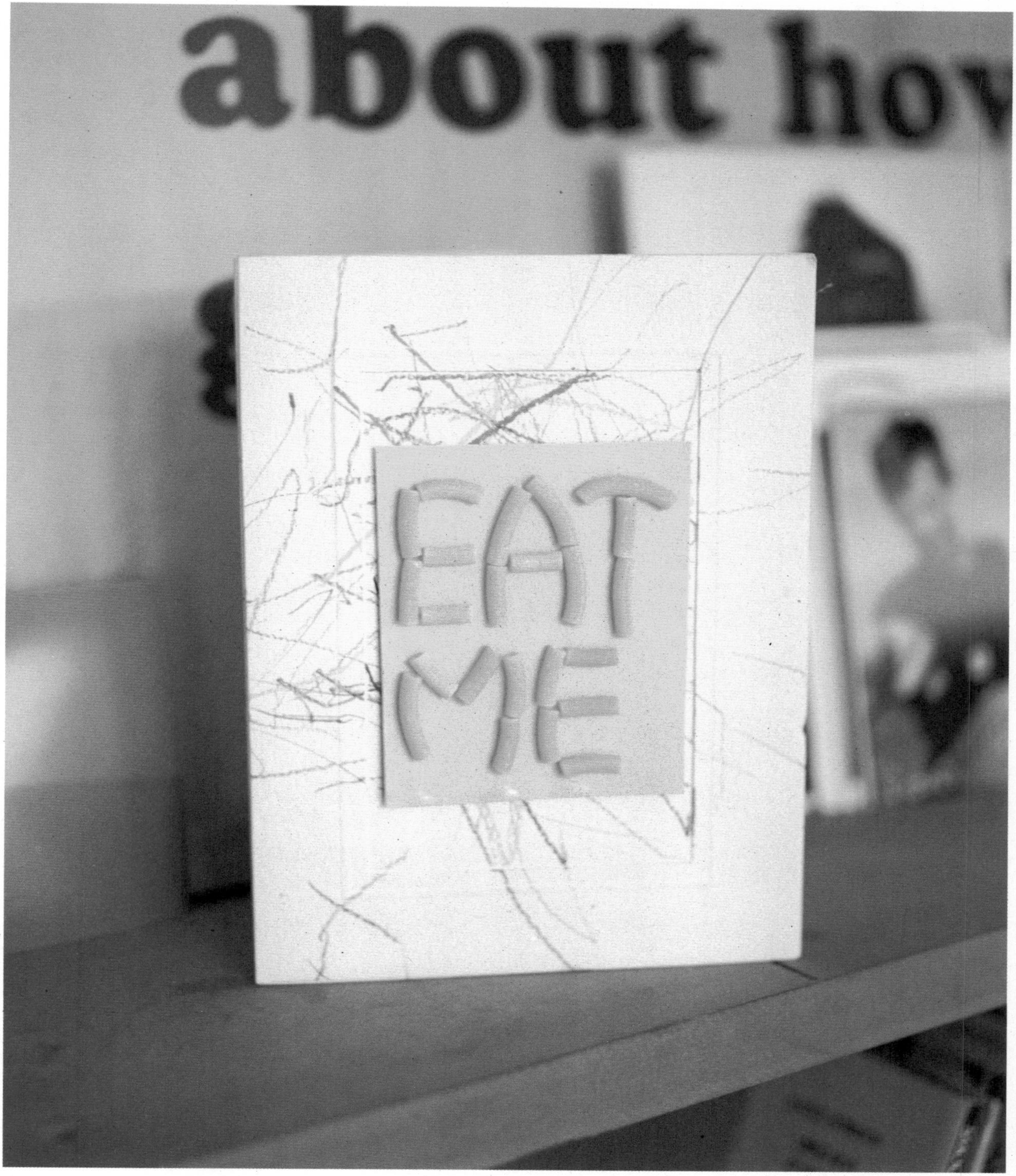
about
EAT
ME

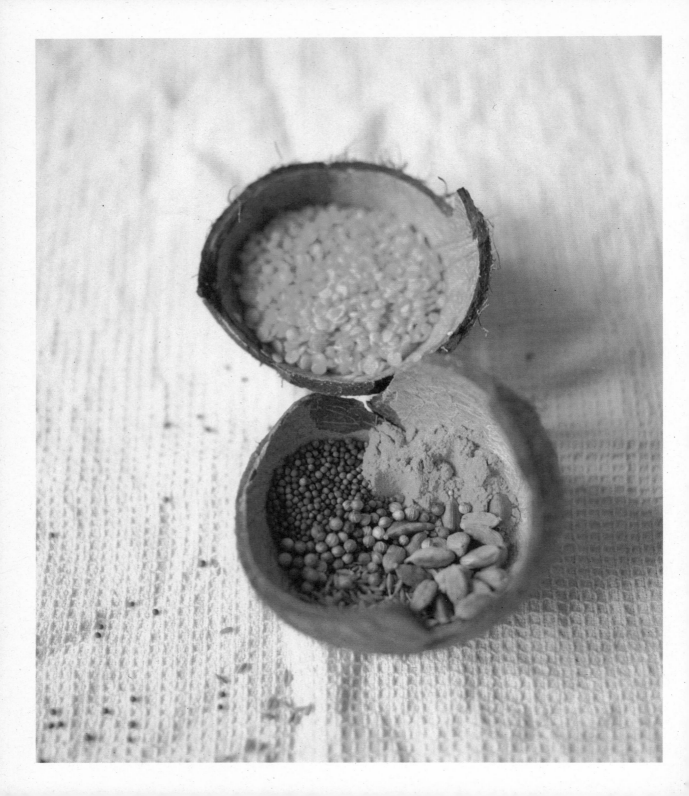

# Quick coconut dhal

Dahl. Daal. Dal. Spicy stuff made using lentils. The charming lady at the Indian High Commission assured us it's 'dal'. Our local curry house (The Kathmandu) reckon it's 'daal'. Our Aslam is adamant you spell it 'dahl'. Who's right? We have no idea.

Serves 6

1 portion of your 5-a-day

olive or groundnut oil

1 red onion, peeled and finely chopped

a small thumb-sized piece of fresh ginger, peeled and finely chopped

1 red chilli, deseeded and finely chopped

2 garlic cloves, peeled and chopped

1 teaspoon yellow mustard seeds

1 teaspoon cumin seeds

1 teaspoon coriander seeds

2 cardamom pods, seeds only

a pinch of turmeric

1 x 400ml tin of coconut milk

500g dried red lentils

1 bay leaf

2 big handfuls of fresh spinach

a small bunch of coriander, stalks removed, leaves roughly chopped

Heat a drizzle of oil in a large saucepan over a low heat and cook the onion, ginger, chilli and garlic for about 10 minutes, until soft.

Meanwhile, grind all the whole spices in a pestle and mortar. Add them to the pan with the turmeric and cook for another couple of minutes.

Next, add the coconut milk, lentils, bay leaf and 1 litre of cold water. Cook for 15 minutes, until the lentils are tender, then stir in the spinach. If the dhal is a little watery, turn up the heat to reduce the sauce down.

Scatter with fresh coriander, and serve with brown rice, a spoonful of yoghurt and a dollop of mango chutney. Or try making the minty yoghurt (page 170) for an extra cooling accompaniment.

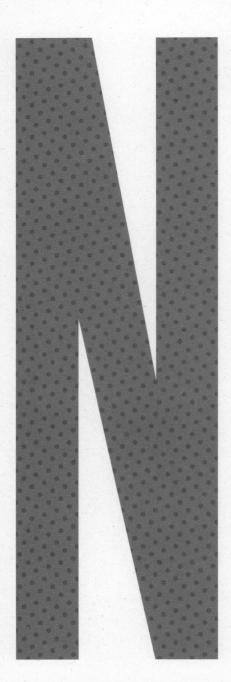

ed the Newt lived around the edge of the pond with his dad, Graham. He had fun with his friends and always did well in school. In fact, you could say that life was pretty perfect for the little lizard apart from one thing – a distinct lack of any exciting food. On the menu most nights was stuff like water-lice risotto, larvae lasagne and (Graham's personal favourite), slug soufflé. As good a chef as his dad was, Ned couldn't help thinking that there was something more – something he hadn't tried yet.

One day on the way to school, Ned came across something he'd never seen before. It was cylindrical in shape and made of glass. It had a wrapper that read 'Hot Curry Paste' and was filled to the brim with a gooey red substance. Checking no one else was around. Ned hid the jar of luminous mystery in a nearby bush and carried on his way to school.

As soon as 3 o'clock rolled around, Ned ran as fast as his adhesive feet would take him to the bush where he had hidden the jar that morning. Glassy-eyed with excitement, he rolled the shiny paste vessel along the muddy path back towards his house. Once inside, Ned hauled the container onto the kitchen table and sat down to inspect his find more closely. After staring at the exotic foodstuff for a while he decided to try and unlock the contents.

But it wouldn't open. After several minutes of wrestling with the jar and not getting anywhere, Ned mustered one last push. 'One, two, THREE!,' he yelled, twisting hard. A loud 'pop' came from the top of the jar. He was in! Ned stuck his snout into the top and was almost knocked off his chair by the pungent aroma that met his newty nostrils. Intrigued, he dipped his lizardy tongue in to get a taste. It was like nothing he had tasted before. Rich, spicy, moreish and, most of all, fiery-hot. He ate the vast majority of the paste very quickly, and soon began to feel rather odd.

Looking down at his feet, Ned noticed that the moist sticky pads he was used to trotting around on were now greener and more scaly than before. He went to inspect his face in the bathroom mirror and saw his once smooth, amphibious features were different. Ned coughed. Smoke came out. 'What's going on?' he thought. He heard a little pop and cocked his head round to look at his back. There, between his little newt shoulders, was a pair of magnificent wings.

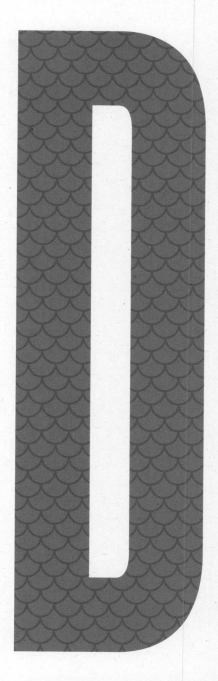

Jumping up excitedly, Ned raced back to the kitchen and grabbed a piece of the drab, newt bread that his dad insisted on buying. He drew in the deepest breath he could muster and exhaled with all his might. A huge flame shot out of his mouth, scorching the bread to a smoking cinder. 'Instant toast!' he exclaimed and began to make piece after piece, dipping his crunchy new invention into what was left of the red paste and munching it down with his new, pointy teeth.

Ned was having so much fun he didn't realise that changing into a dragon and cremating lots of bread had taken quite a long time, and that his dad would soon be home. He continued to fly around, stroke his new scales and practise his fire breathing, completely oblivious of the time, until suddenly his dad appeared at the door.

'Ned! What on earth is going on?' Graham exclaimed, placing a sticky foot on the jar. 'Um, I found this paste and may have tried a little bit of it,' came the meek reply. 'A bit?' cried his dad, 'Look at you, you're a dragon! Luckily you haven't turned enormous yet, which can be another unfortunate by-product of newts coming into contact with hot food.'

'Wait a minute,' said Ned, 'How do you know that newts turn into dragons when they eat hot food?' 'Because, Ned my boy, exactly the same thing happened to me when I was a lad,' Graham explained. 'Unfortunately, I wasn't so lucky – I grew to 400 times my normal size. Your granddad wasn't too pleased with the state of the kitchen ceiling, I can tell you. Then again, I was eating raw chillies.'

'Well, how do I change back?' asked Ned. 'As much fun as this is, I don't think I'll be allowed back in school if there's even a remote chance of fire coming out of my nostrils.' Graham smiled. 'Well...' he said, 'It's actually pretty easy. All you've got to do is eat something else to counteract the hotness of the paste – a nice slug soufflé should do it!'

Ned might have had to turn into a dragon to find out, but he finally understood why he and his dad ate what they did. Newts and hot food just don't mix. Luckily, you're not a newt, so don't be afraid of experimenting with foods that have a bit of a kick. Plus, if you do sprout a pair of wings after a curry or a nice spot of chilli, then it means you must be part newt. Which we think would actually be quite cool. The En

# Squash, tomato and chickpea curry

**In a hurry to make this curry? No need to peel. Just chop, squash and let it bubble away.**

Bash the mustard and fennel seeds in a pestle and mortar.

Heat a drizzle of olive oil in a big pan over a medium heat and cook the onion, garlic and chilli for about 10 minutes, until soft. Add the curry leaves or powder, coriander and ground mustard and fennel seeds and cook for another couple of minutes.

Next, add the squash, lime juice and honey and cook for a minute or so. Squash in the cherry tomatoes using your hands, then add the tinned tomatoes, drained chickpeas and coconut milk and simmer for 20 minutes, until the squash is cooked through.

About 10 minutes before serving, pop the flatbreads into the oven on a low heat.

Season the curry and serve with the warm flatbreads, a dollop of plain yoghurt and a few sprigs of coriander. For an extra-cooling yoghurt, try the minty version on page 170.

Serves 4
3 portions of your 5-a-day

1 teaspoon mustard seeds
1 teaspoon fennel seeds
olive oil
1 red onion, peeled and finely sliced
2 garlic cloves, peeled and finely chopped
1 green chilli, deseeded and finely chopped
a few curry leaves or 1 teaspoon curry powder
a small bunch of coriander, stalks removed, leaves finely chopped
1 medium butternut squash, peeled and cut into medium chunks
juice of 2 limes
a drizzle of honey
2 handfuls of cherry tomatoes
1 x 400g tin of tomatoes
1 x 400g tin of chickpeas, drained and rinsed
1 x 400ml tin of coconut milk

To serve
4 flatbreads
4 tablespoons plain yoghurt
a few sprigs of fresh coriander

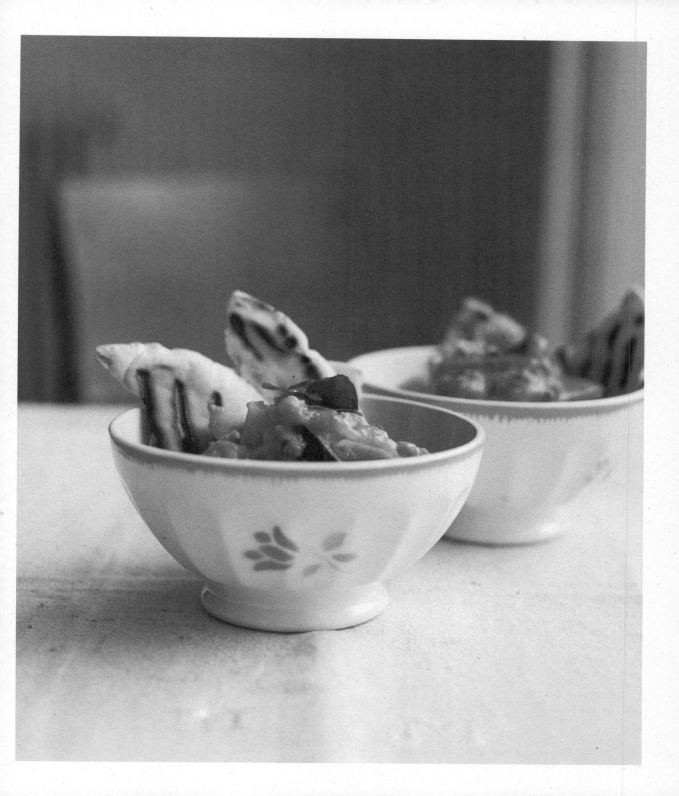

# Sweet potato beanie bake

There's more veg in this vegetable bake than you can shake a very large stick at, so no need to faff about with rice or pasta. Just a green salad and you're good to go.

Serves 4
3 portions of your 5-a-day

olive oil
2 red onions, peeled and
    finely sliced
2 garlic cloves, peeled and
    finely sliced
2 carrots, peeled and finely
    chopped
1 teaspoon smoked paprika
2 sweet potatoes, scrubbed
    and cut into medium chunks
2 bay leaves
2 sprigs of thyme
1 x 400g tin of chopped
    tomatoes
1 x 400g tin of butter beans,
    drained and rinsed
1 x 400g tin of cannellini or
    borlotti beans, drained and
    rinsed

For the breadcrumb topping
2 slices of stale or oven-dried
    bread
a small bunch of flat-leaf
    parsley, leaves picked
zest of 1 lemon

Preheat your oven to 200°C/400°F/gas mark 6.

Heat a splash of olive oil in a big pan and cook the onions, garlic and carrots for 5 to 10 minutes, until soft. Stir in the smoked paprika and cook for another minute or so.

Add the sweet potatoes and a mugful (about 200ml) of water, then turn down the heat and allow to simmer until the potatoes are almost cooked and most of the water has evaporated.

Stir in the herbs, tomatoes and drained beans and bring to the boil.

While this is cooking, put the stale bread, parsley and lemon zest into a food processor and whizz to fine breadcrumbs. If you don't have a food processor, put the bread into a sandwich bag and bash to breadcrumbs, then finely chop the parsley leaves and mix with the lemon zest.

Pour the bean mixture into an ovenproof casserole dish, cover with the breadcrumb topping, drizzle with olive oil and bake for 15 minutes, until bubbling and golden brown on top.

Serve with a big green salad.

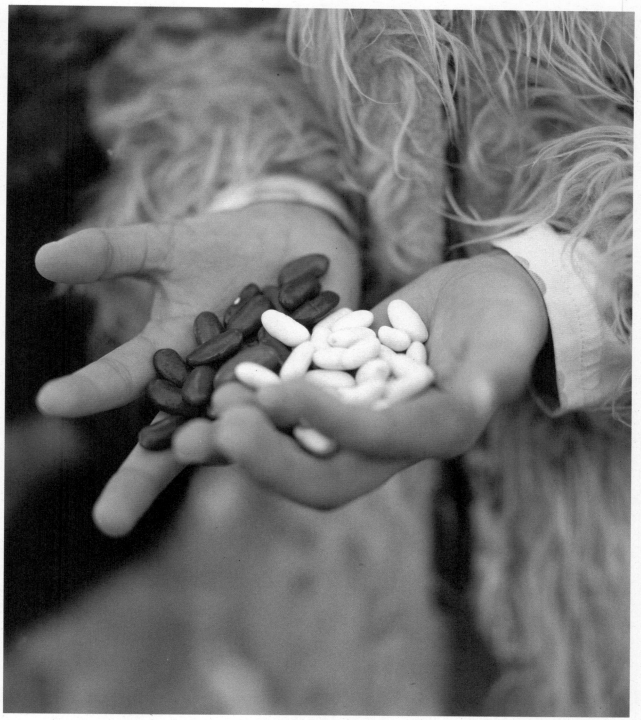

'I keep the red ones in my right pocket, the white ones in the left, and the green ones in my inside pocket, with my biros.'

# Eggy rice

Rice is nice but eggy rice is even better. Especially when it comes with a little chilli kick.

Peel and finely chop the ginger and garlic, finely slice the spring onions and pak choi, and grate the carrot. Set all these aside.

Put a wok or a big frying pan over a high heat and let it get really hot. Add a splash of groundnut oil and lightly scramble the beaten eggs for about a minute. When just cooked through, remove the eggs from the pan and drain on some kitchen roll.

Give the wok or pan a clean and add a splash more oil. Add the onion, ginger and garlic and fry for a couple of minutes, until they start to colour up. Then stir in the honey and rice wine and cook for another minute.

Now add the cooked rice, scrambled egg, spring onions, pak choi, carrot, oyster sauce, a splash of sesame oil, juice of 1 lime and a big glug of soy sauce.

Turn up the heat and cook for 5 more minutes, until the rice is piping hot.

Serve with a wedge of lime and a dash of chilli sauce for an extra kick.

# Cheddar pie

Pies were originally invented to transport the stuff inside. Sort of like edible Tupperware. Back in the days before colour telly, some even had small orchestras and jesters inside to liven up royal banquets. This one is a bit of a treat which contains that winning combination of cheese, leeks and potatoes (we left out the variety show).

Serves 8

counts towards your 5-a-day

100g potatoes, peeled and
    cut into little chunks
a knob of butter
1 large onion, peeled and
    finely chopped
1 big leek, washed, trimmed
    and finely sliced
150g mature Cheddar cheese,
    grated
4 tablespoons milk
a few sprigs of thyme or
    rosemary, stalks removed
3 large free-range eggs
1 x 500g pack of ready-made
    puff pastry (for a lighter
    version, try using half a
    packet and making a lattice
    or one of the shapes on
    page 136)

Preheat the oven to 190°C/375°F/gas mark 5. You'll need a shallow tart tin about 20cm diameter for this recipe.

Put the potatoes into a big pan, cover with boiling water and bring to the boil. Simmer for 6 to 8 minutes, until just cooked through.

While the spuds are boiling, melt the butter in a pan and fry the onion and leek until soft. Set aside to cool.

Drain the potatoes, allow to cool a little, then mix in the onion, leek, cheese, milk, herbs and 2 of the eggs. Beat the other egg in a bowl, ready for the pastry.

Dust a clean work surface with flour. Using a rolling pin, roll out two-thirds of the puff pastry until it's a few centimetres bigger than the tart tin and roughly the thickness of a pound coin. Roll the pastry round the rolling pin and drape it over the top of the tart tin. Use your fingers to press it into the sides of the tin and allow the edges to overhang a little.

Tip the cheese and onion mixture into the middle and spread out. Flip the edges back over and brush with some of the beaten egg.

Roll out the remaining pastry to the same thickness and lay it over the top of the pie. Snip off any excess and pinch the edges together with your fingers. Brush the whole pie with the rest of the beaten egg and bake in the oven for 45 minutes, until golden brown.

Serve with lightly buttered peas or steamed broccoli.

# PIE SYMBOLOGY 101

## Or 'How to win friends and influence people using the little pastry decoration on top of your pie'

Whether it be a belated birthday present, a declaration of love or a reminder to renew the car insurance, if you've got something important to tell someone, simply bake them a nice pie. Fashion one of the symbols below and let the baked goods do the talking. Say it with love, say with malice but above all, say it with pastry.

I'm cheerful. Or I baked this for the Sun God Ra

Dear pie recipient, I love you

Dear pie recipient, I know about Barbara

There's trouble in Gotham

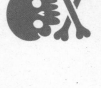

I was at Woodstock and in many ways, still am

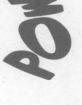

This pie is to be enjoyed only at my house

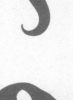

Pie from the sky

There's a melting clock in this pie

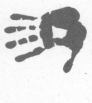

Superpie

Birthday pie

Cool guys make pies

They'd run out of turkeys

My first pie

Made by my own fair hands

We be pie-rates

# QUICK LATTICE GUIDE

Congratulations on your new fridge/freezer

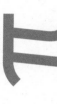

Rainy day pie

We're having a picnic, and we're taking this pie

Tastier than 3.14

Pieeeeeeeeee

My theatre career is going well. Celebratory pie

I'm still waiting for my Equity card. Annoyed pie

I hail from Texas

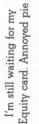

I've made good use of leftovers

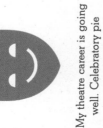

You will let me have the last piece of this pie

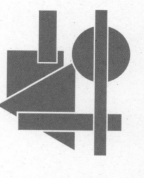

I outgrew lattice in the 80s. My pie is a savoury tribute to Kandinsky

I am very bad at lattice. In fact, I don't think this really counts at all

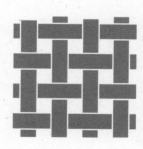

I am good at lattice. My pie is secure, pretty and breathable

# Roasted root veg

**Roasty, rooty and really rather good.**

Serves 4 (with leftovers)
2½ portions of your 5-a-day

For the veg
1 butternut squash
2 large fresh beetroots
2 parsnips
6 carrots
8 garlic cloves
a few sprigs of thyme
olive oil

For the dressing
a small bunch of mint
1 tablespoon red wine
    vinegar
2 tablespoons honey
½ a red chilli, finely chopped
4 tablespoons olive oil

To serve
plain yoghurt
a handful of toasted pumpkin
    seeds
bread, toasted

Preheat your oven to 200°C/400°F/gas mark 6.

Top and tail the squash, then cut it in half and scoop out the seeds. Slice it into chunky strips lengthways. You can leave the skin on for this, as it tastes wonderful roasted. Give the rest of the veg a good scrub, then top and tail them. Cut the beetroots and parsnips into quarters and the carrots in half lengthways.

Put all the veg into a big roasting tray with the garlic cloves (no need to peel them). Add the thyme, drizzle with olive oil and season well. Toss the whole lot together until the veg are lightly coated, then put the tray into the oven and roast them for 50 minutes, until golden.

While the veg are roasting, make the dressing. Finely chop the mint and mix it in a bowl with the rest of the ingredients.

Once the veg are ready, take them out of the oven and remove the garlic cloves from the tray. Let the garlic cool a little, then squeeze it out of its skins into the dressing. Mix well, then pour the dressing over the roast veg and give everything a good stir.

Serve a pile of roast veg topped with a couple of spoonfuls of yoghurt, a scattering of pumpkin seeds and some toasted bread to mop it all up with.

For extra veg, add a simple rocket or leafy salad. A little sprinkling of crumbled feta or goat's cheese works really well too.

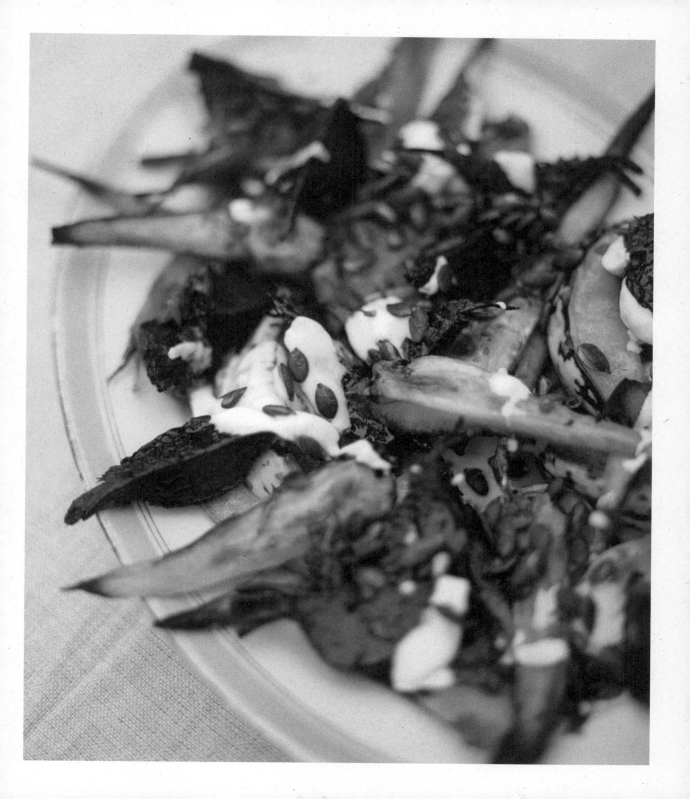

# IT'S A CONUNDRUM

Harry Pearce is a man who likes the alphabet. He also likes puzzles. So in a very clever move, he's combined the two to make these conundrums. There are ten phrases hidden amongst these words and letters. Find them all to claim the title of King or Queen Alphabet for the rest of the year. All will bow down at your superior feet. Answers at the end of the book.

1

# FREUDIAN

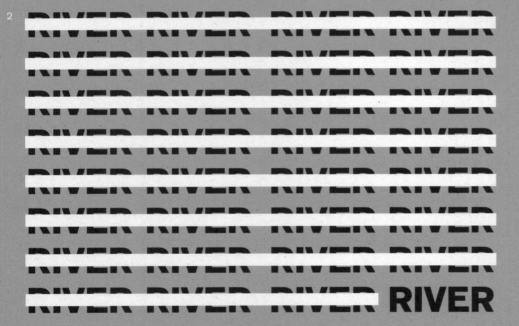

2

RIVER RIVER RIVER RIVER
RIVER RIVER RIVER RIVER
RIVER RIVER RIVER RIVER
RIVER RIVER RIVER RIVER
RIVER RIVER RIVER RIVER
RIVER RIVER RIVER RIVER
RIVER RIVER RIVER RIVER
RIVER RIVER RIVER RIVER

3

**HEART**
**HAND**

4 **RNOAD**

5

ILNOOK
ABNAGCE
KR

6

SMOKE

SMOKE

SMOKESMOKE

7

HERE
THERE

8

SYMPHON

9

EGGS
EGGS
EGGS
EGGS
EGGS
EGGS

SHOP

10

# GOOD THINGS TO HAVE FOR DINNER

---

# FISH

# CATCH

For as long as we've been near the sea, us humans have been eating fish. But over-fishing, damaging methods and failing policies mean that many species are under threat and others are dying needlessly. At the moment, 50% of all fish caught in the North Sea are thrown back dead – either because the catch is over quota or because the fishermen can't sell it.

So if you want your grandchildren's grandkids to enjoy a good stargazy pie, we need to start buying responsibly, and now.

The more sustainable fish aren't as famous or widely available as something like cod, so it will take some willpower and effort to seek them out. But to help improve things for our scaled friends, you can also start making a fuss by asking where the fish on offer came from and how it was caught. The more our supermarkets and local fishmongers hear this sort of stuff, the more likely they'll be to start sourcing responsibly, the more likely they are to start stocking unusual species and the more likely it is that our seas will start to recover.

Here's a list of the top fish to seek out. They're in plentiful supply, are caught in a sustainable manner and are worth searching for:

Sprats, pollack (a good swap for cod), pouting, mackerel (ideally line-caught), trout (again, line-caught is best), megrim, witch, scad (or horse mackerel), black bream (swap for bass, especially those from Cornwall, the North West and North Wales), grey mullet, red gurnard, garfish, rainbow trout (organic or freshwater farmed) and lemon sole (which is a good substitute for Dover sole).

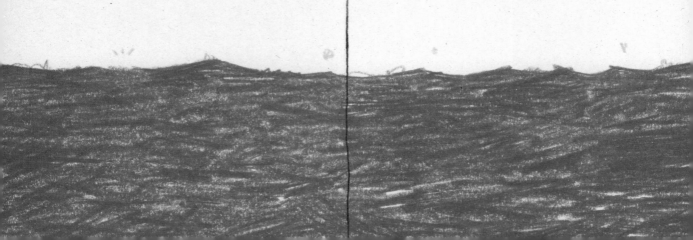

# RELEASE

And here's the list of fish to eat less frequently. Or better still, leave them alone for a few years to up their numbers. If in doubt, have a look at the Marine Conservation Society's website www.fishonline.org for advice on which sustainable sea food to buy.

Whitebait, cod from the Atlantic or UK (unless MSC-certified or organically farmed), haddock (except line-caught, Icelandic), plaice, hake, bluefin tuna, sharks and huss, skate and rays (unless self-caught, line-caught and tagged, or organically farmed), wild salmon, tropical prawns, halibut (except farmed onshore), brown or sea trout and eel.

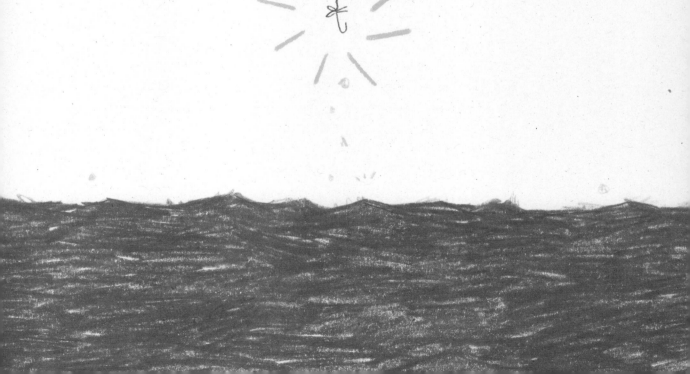

# One mean, green fish pie

If this pie was a person, it would live in a little pebble-dashed cottage overlooking some cliffs, know all the words to 'Haul Away Joe' and have a fine collection of navy cable-knit jumpers.

Serves 4–6
2 portions of your 5-a-day

For the pie bit
500ml milk
1 bay leaf
a sprinkling of peppercorns
100g butter
2 leeks, washed, trimmed and
    finely sliced
2 tablespoons plain flour
400g white fish (line-caught
    Icelandic haddock or
    pollack), cut into chunks
200g undyed smoked fish
    fillets (haddock, rainbow or
    freshwater trout)
3 large handfuls of spinach
freshly grated nutmeg

For the pea mash
600g floury potatoes,
    quartered
300g frozen peas
extra virgin olive oil
a knob of butter
a few sprigs of mint, chopped

To serve
2 lemons

Preheat your oven to 200°C/400°F/gas mark 6.

Put the milk, bay leaf and peppercorns into a pan over a low heat and allow to simmer for 5 minutes. Then remove from the heat, take out the bay leaf and peppercorns, and set to one side.

Melt half the butter in a large casserole. Add the leeks and cook until soft, then set aside.

Place the potatoes in a large pan of boiling water and bring back to the boil. Reduce the heat and leave to simmer for 10 minutes.

Meanwhile, add the remaining butter to the softened leeks. When it has melted, stir in the flour and cook for a couple of minutes, until the sauce starts to thicken. Gradually add the milk, continuing to stir the leek mixture and removing any lumps with the back of a wooden spoon. Once all the milk has been incorporated, add the fish, spinach and a good grating of nutmeg. Stir well and take off the heat.

The potatoes should have had about 10 minutes by this point, so add the peas and simmer for another few minutes, until the potatoes are cooked. Drain the potatoes and peas in a colander and allow to drip dry, then chuck them back into the pan. Drizzle in some olive oil, add a knob of butter, sprinkle in the mint and season well before giving them a good mashing.

Pile the pea mash on top of the fish mixture, even it out with the back of a fork and pop the casserole into the oven for 25 minutes, until golden brown.

Serve in big scoops, with steamed green beans and lemon wedges.

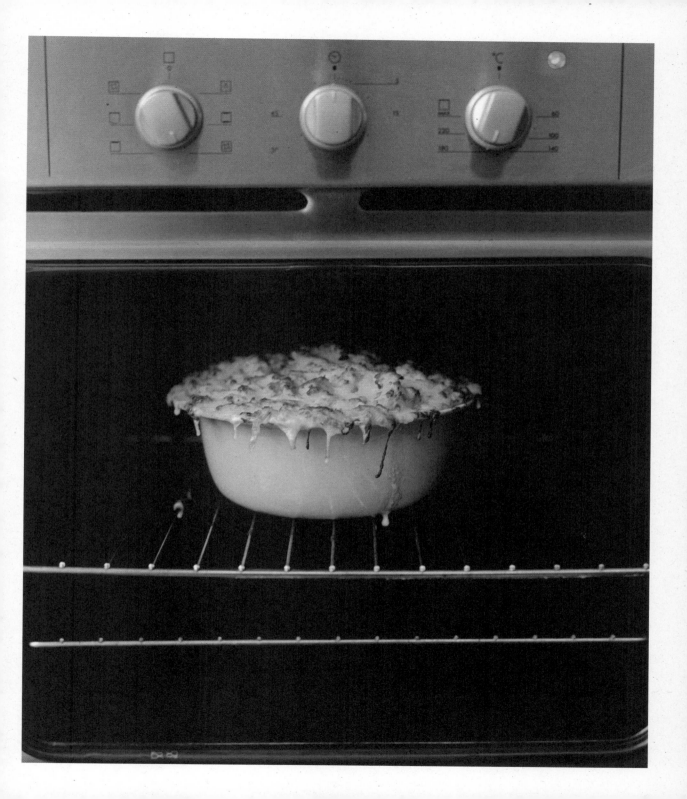

# Hearty fishcakes

**Gurnard, pollack and coley work just as well for this recipe.**

counts towards your 5-a-day

500g Maris Piper or good
    mashing potatoes, peeled
150g broccoli
600g boneless, skinless
    sustainable salmon fillets
olive oil
a few sprigs of parsley,
    leaves picked and roughly
    chopped
zest of 1 lemon
2 slices of wholemeal bread
    (slightly stale – a couple of
    days old is best)
2 free-range eggs, beaten
2 tablespoons plain flour

Cut the potatoes into little chunks, put them into a pan, cover with boiling water and simmer for 5 minutes. While the spuds are cooking, chop up the broccoli into florets. When the potatoes have been cooking for 5 minutes, chuck the broccoli in.

Rub the salmon with a drizzle of olive oil. If you've got a steamer, put the fish into one of the colander layers and place it on top of the spuds. If not, a metal colander works just as well. Put a lid on top and leave to steam for about 7 minutes, or until the fish is cooked.

Once the potatoes are done and the fish is just cooked, take the whole lot off the heat. Drain the potatoes and broccoli in a colander and allow to dry off completely, then put back into the pan and mash. Let the salmon cool completely, then flake into the mash. Add the parsley leaves and lemon zest. Mix well and season.

If you've got a food processor, whizz up the bread into fine breadcrumbs. Alternatively, dry it out in the oven on a low heat, cool, then pop into a plastic bag and give it a good bash with a rolling pin.

Beat the eggs in a bowl, put the breadcrumbs on one plate and the flour on to another. Place in a row, starting with flour, then the egg mixture and ending with the breadcrumbs.

Shape the mixture into 4 big cakes or 8 smaller ones, depending on who you are feeding. Then dip each fishcake into the flour, then into the egg and finally roll them around in the breadcrumbs until well coated. If you're going to freeze them, do this now, wrapping them in clingfilm first. Otherwise, pop into the fridge for 30 minutes to firm up.

Preheat the oven to 200°C/400°F/gas mark 6. Place the fishcakes on a baking tray, lightly drizzle with olive oil and bake in the oven for 10 minutes. Then flip them over and bake for another 10 minutes, until golden brown on both sides.

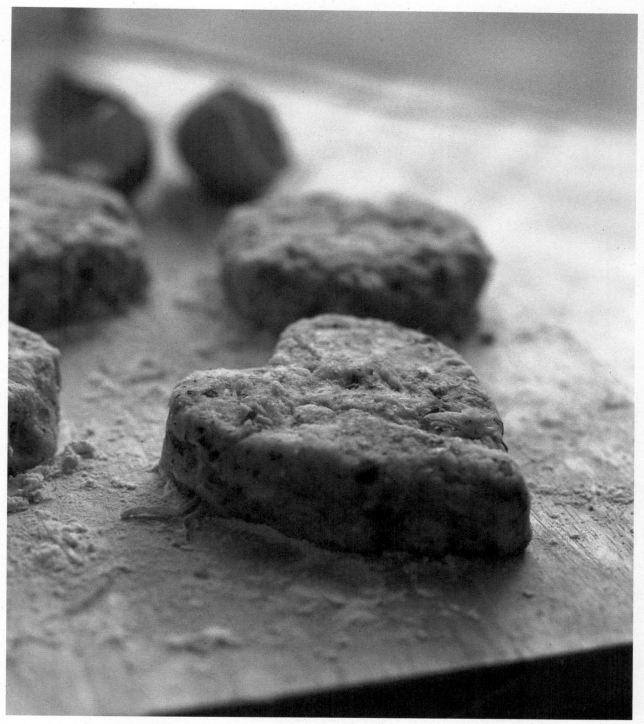

Serve with rainbow chips (page 224), a green salad (page 211) and a side of galoshes.

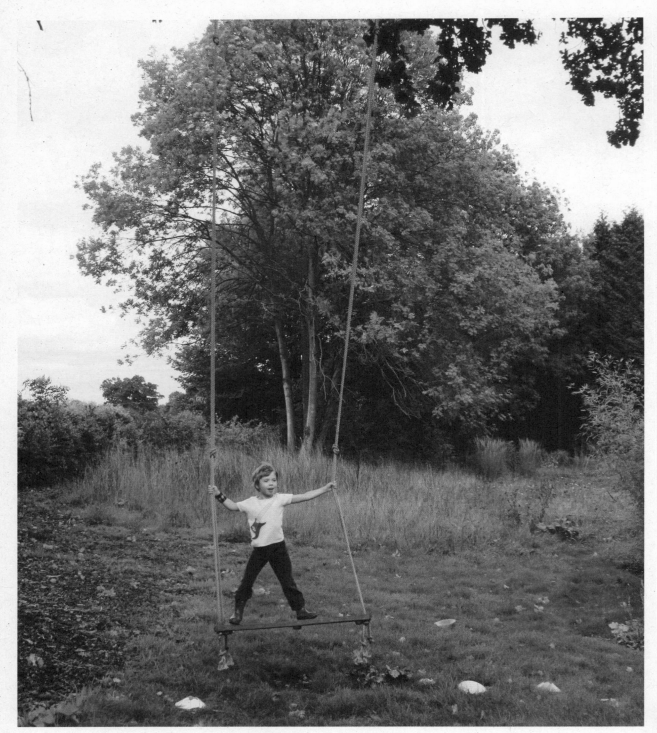

(No actual coconut trees pictured)

# Coconut fish curry

2½ portions of your 5-a-day

**For the curry**
olive oil
1 red onion, peeled and finely
    chopped
2 garlic cloves, peeled and
    finely chopped
a small knob of fresh ginger,
    peeled and finely chopped
2 tablespoons garam masala
1 x 400g tin of coconut milk
1 x 400g tin of chopped
    tomatoes
500g fish fillets, skinned,
    boned and cut into chunks
    (sustainably caught salmon,
    white fish like pollack or
    line-caught haddock work
    really well)
a large handful of sugarsnap
    peas
2 handfuls of fresh spinach

**For the cucumber yoghurt**
½ a cucumber, finely grated
6 tablespoons plain yoghurt
juice of 1 lime
a few sprigs of mint, stalks
    removed and leaves roughly
    chopped

Three amazing things you might not know about coconuts:

- The clear liquid inside can also be used as a blood plasma substitute.
- You're 10 times more likely to be hit by a falling coconut than attacked by a shark.
- Coconuts can power factories (the one we get our coconut milk from runs on old coconut shells. Which is as sustainable as it gets).

This hairy fruit also goes rather well with fish. That's why we've included it in this recipe. Technically, that's four things but the last one was sort of obvious.

Heat a little olive oil in a wok or a big frying pan and cook the onion, garlic and ginger for 5 to 10 minutes, until soft.

Add the garam masala and cook for another minute, then add the coconut milk and tomatoes. Turn down the heat and allow to simmer for 10 minutes or so, until the sauce starts to thicken.

Add the fish pieces, the sugarsnap peas and spinach. Simmer away for 5 minutes or so, until the fish turns opaque and starts to flake.

Meanwhile, mix the grated cucumber, yoghurt, lime juice and chopped mint in a bowl.

Serve the fish curry in bowls, with brown basmati, the cucumber yoghurt and a few grilled poppadoms. If you want to spice things up, sprinkle some chopped red chillies on top.

# Prawn phad thai

Along with the obligatory wooden elephants, those triangle chair-cushion things and a taste for spicy shredded papaya, this is probably the tastiest thing we picked up from Thailand. You can use chicken breast or tofu instead of the prawns. Same same but different.

Serves 4
counts towards your 5-a-day

For the phad thai
200g rice noodles (we like the big flat ones best)
2 tablespoons tamarind paste
2 tablespoons fish sauce
1 tablespoon honey
juice of 2 limes
4 tablespoons peanuts, roasted in the oven or dry roasted in a pan
groundnut oil
2 garlic cloves, peeled and finely chopped
1 red chilli, deseeded and finely chopped
4 spring onions, finely sliced
12 raw peeled big prawns, heads removed
2 large free-range eggs
2 carrots, peeled and grated
2 handfuls of beansprouts
a big bunch of coriander, stalks removed
2 limes

Put the noodles in a bowl and cover with boiling water. Leave for about 15 minutes, or according to the packet directions, until softened.

Mix the tamarind paste with 2 tablespoons of boiling water and mix well. Add the fish sauce, honey and lime juice, stir well and set aside.

Use a pestle and mortar to grind up the roasted peanuts, and pop them into a bowl for later.

Once your noodles are ready, drain them and use scissors to cut them into manageable lengths (get a grown up to help). Then deal with everything that needs chopping, grating or slicing.

Now place a wok or a big frying pan over a high heat until really hot and starting to smoke. Add a good splash of oil and quickly fry the garlic, chilli and spring onions for a minute or so. Add the prawns and cook for another few minutes, until they turn from grey to pink.

Crack in the eggs and let them cook without breaking them up for a couple of minutes. Then add the drained noodles and give everything a proper stir for another minute or so, making sure no egg sticks to the bottom of the pan.

Pour in the tamarind mixture and cook for another 2 minutes, then add the carrots, beansprouts, a sprinkling of the crushed peanuts and half the coriander. Stir for a minute, then remove from the heat.

Serve your phad thai in bowls, sprinkled generously with the rest of the crushed peanuts and coriander, and with the remaining 2 limes, cut into wedges, alongside.

# Fish in a little bag, Sicilian style

Forget boil-in-the-bag kippers. This Sicilian-inspired healthy meal-in-a-bag works really well with any fillet of fish and won't make your house smell like a 1950s B&B.

Serves 4

counts towards your 5-a-day

300g quinoa
2 handfuls of cherry tomatoes, quartered
300ml hot chicken or vegetable stock
a pinch of ground cinnamon
1 lemon
a small bunch of basil, stalks removed
4 x 150g fillets of your favourite fish, skinned and boned

Preheat your oven to 200°C/400°F/gas mark 6.

Put the quinoa into a pan with the tomatoes, stock and a pinch of cinnamon. Bring to the boil and simmer for 10 minutes.

To make each bag, take a large piece of kitchen foil (roughly the size of 2 A4 sheets) and fold it in half. Fold over the 2 sides several times to make a little bag, leaving the top open. Then place on a baking tray.

Take the quinoa off the heat and cover with a lid till all the water is absorbed. Then finely grate the lemon zest into the quinoa and tear in the basil. Mix well and divide between the 4 bags. Chop the lemon into wedges.

Place a piece of fish on top of each pile of quinoa mix, season with salt and pepper, then top with a couple of lemon wedges and seal up the bags.

Bake in the oven for 20 to 25 minutes, until the fish is opaque and cooked through. Serve with a green salad (page 211).

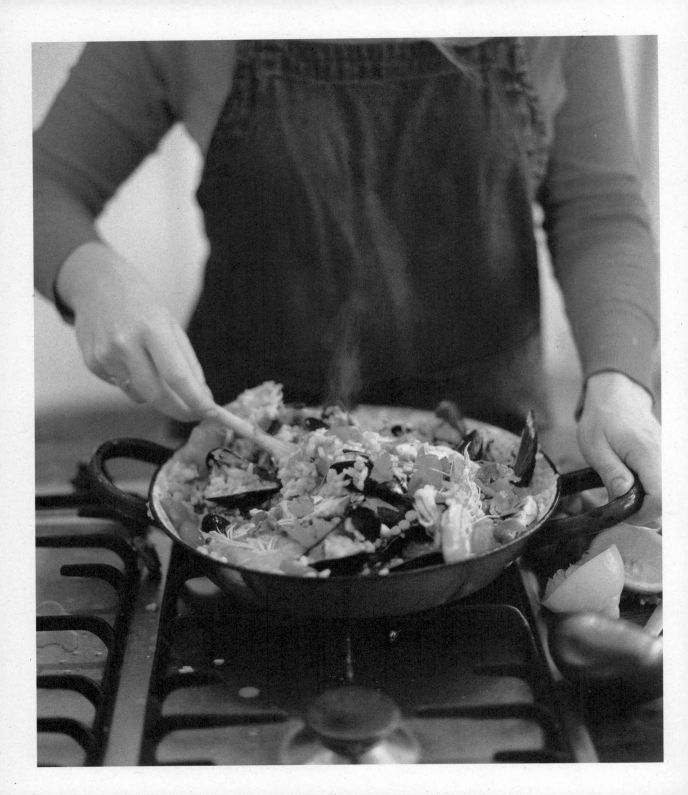

# Paella

Prawns, mussels, clams, crispy chicken, chorizo, peas, tomatoes – it's a one-pan dinner with a bit of everything in it. Simply leave out any bits you're not keen on or just chuck the whole lot into the mix. You'll need to use your biggest casserole pan or stock pot for this recipe (and keep a beady eye on it to ensure the rice doesn't stick).

Preheat your oven to 180°C/350°F/gas mark 4.

Dust the chicken with flour, salt and pepper and fry them in a little olive oil in a large pan until golden brown all over. Then cut into strips, place on a baking tray and pop into the bottom of the oven while you get on with everything else.

Place the pan on a medium heat and fry the chorizo and bacon until crispy. Add the onion and garlic and cook for 5 to 10 minutes, until soft. Pour in half the stock, add the saffron and heat till bubbling.

Once bubbling, add the rice and leave to cook for about 20 minutes on a low heat, stirring occasionally to stop the rice sticking. Add a little more stock if needed.

After 20 minutes, the rice should be nearly cooked (it needs a bit of bite – not too mushy, not filling-inducing). Add the rest of the stock, the peas, prawns, mussels and/or clams, and squid and stir well.

Squash the tomatoes into the pan with your hands, then cover and cook for 10 minutes.

Once the prawns have turned pink and the mussels and clams have opened, make sure the rice is properly cooked and turn off the heat. Discard any unopened clams and mussels, then add the chicken strips, which should be cooked and crispy by now. Squeeze half a lemon over the top, scatter with chopped parsley and serve with the rest of the lemons, cut into wedges.

Serves 6
1 portion of your 5-a-day

6 skin-on boneless free-range chicken breasts or thighs
plain flour, for dusting
olive oil
100g cooking chorizo (make sure it's the softer chorizo used for cooking, not the cured salami sort), chopped
6 slices of streaky bacon, chopped
1 onion, peeled and chopped
4 garlic cloves, peeled and finely sliced
2 litres chicken stock
2 large pinches of saffron
500g paella rice
2 handfuls of peas, fresh or frozen
6 big king prawns (shell on)
500g mussels and/or clams, well scrubbed
2 small squid, cleaned and cut into bite-sized rings
2 handfuls of cherry tomatoes
2 lemons
a small bunch of flat-leaf parsley, stalks removed

# THINGS TO DO IN  Minutes

While you're waiting for things to rise

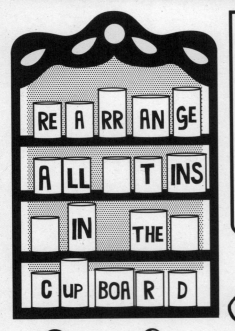

REARRANGE ALL TINS IN THE CUPBOARD

*Write your shopping list*

## SET THE DINNER TABLE

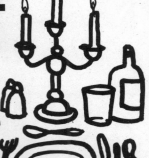

MAKE DIP EAT DIP

**WASH** YOUR DOG / CAT / BROTHER

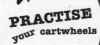

**PRACTISE** your cartwheels

PLANT FLOWERS SEEDS HERBS

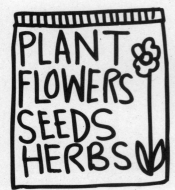

DESCALE THE KETTLE FILL WITH VINEGAR THEN BOIL — RINSE

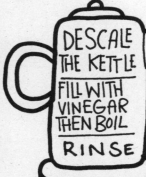

SOCK SK8

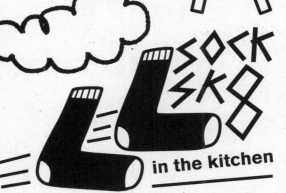

in the kitchen

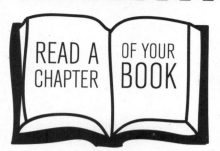

READ A CHAPTER OF YOUR BOOK

PLOT APRIL FOOLS

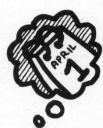

MAKE A WELCOME SIGN FOR YOUR HOUSE

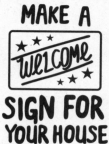

BIRO TATTOO

GO ROUND THE HOUSE AND NAME ANYTHING AND EVERYTHING THAT'S IN A FRAMED PICTURE ON A WALL

**15 MINUTE NATURAL (AND TASTY) SOOTHING FACE MASK**

Mash up a ripe banana, add a cup of porridge oats, and mix it all up. Add enough milk to create a nice paste. Apply the oatmeal and banana paste to your face and leave it on for about 10 minutes. Then rinse off.

BUBBLES

BUBBLES

BUBBLES

BUBBLES

LEARN A MAGIC TRICK

MAKE AFTERNOON TEA. WITH CUPS AND SAUCERS AND EVERYTHING

MAKE A PLAYING CARD TOWER

DIG WEEDS

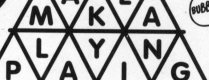

Invent a cure for hiccups

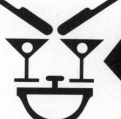

MAKE FACES FROM UTENSILS

# GOOD THINGS TO HAVE FOR DINNER

---

# MEAT

# HAVE A BUTCHER'S

If you're looking for a cut above the rest, then your best bet is a trip to your local butcher. Yes, we know it's the obvious and 'officially correct' thing to say but you'll get far more out of having a chinwag with your butcher than simply knowing where your meat has come from.

They'll be able to tell you exactly how to cook whatever you buy, can suggest other stuff to make with it (and serve it with) and might even chuck in a sausage if you're nice. So you don't look like a plum when you go in there, here's a simple guide to what's what in the world of meat.

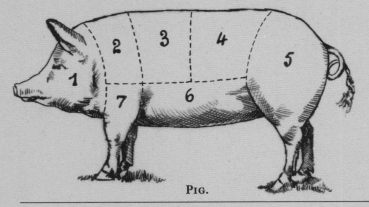

PIG.

1. BRAWN. 2. NECK. 3. LOIN PORK. 4. RUMP PORK. 5. LEG PORK. 6. BELLY. 7. HAND.

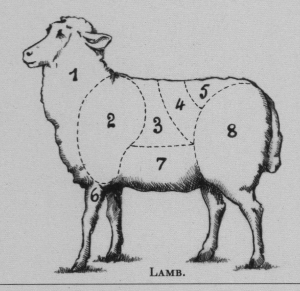

LAMB.

1. NECK. 2. SHOULDER. 3. RACK. 4. LOIN. 5. CHUMP. 6. SHANK. 7. BREAST. 8. LEG.

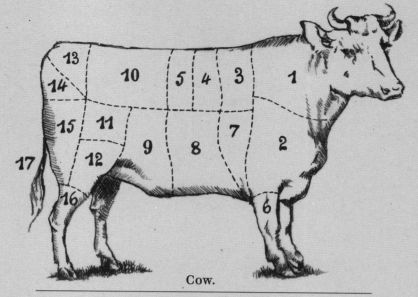

**Cow.**

1. Sticken. 2. Clod. 3. Chuck Steak. 4. Middle Ribs. 5. Fore Ribs. 6. Shin. 7. Shoulder.
8. Brisket. 9. Thin Flank. 10. Sirloin T-bones. 11. Veiny Piece. 12. Thick Flank. 13. Rump Steak.
14. Topside. 15. Round. 16. Leg. 17. Oxtail.

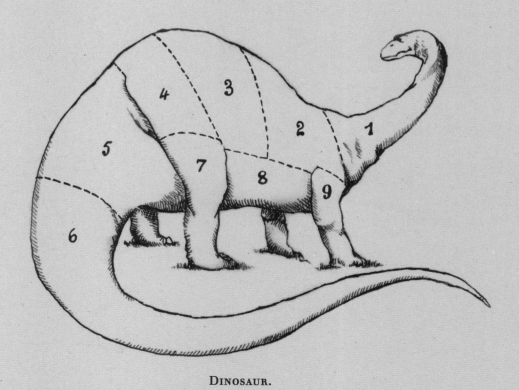

**Dinosaur.**

1. Neck-for-a-month. 2. Fred Flintstone's driving seat. 3. Good vantage point. 4. Jurassic steak.
5. Rumpasaurus. 6. Completely Enormous Tail. 7. BBQ for 400. 8. The Belly ot the Beast. 9. BBQ for 385.

# Sausage and squash mash

Given that 2 apples, a butternut squash and a couple of sweet potatoes are unlikely to break the bank (plus you'll probably already have stuff like honey and mustard in your cupboard), it's definitely worth forking out for some top-quality bangers here. As long as you've got good sausages and a decent potato masher, the rest will be easy.

Preheat your oven to 200°C/400°F/gas mark 6.

Put the sausages into a baking tray and add the apple wedges.

Mix the mustard, honey and apple juice together in a small bowl, then pour over the sausages and apples and give it a good stir.

Bake in the oven for 20 to 25 minutes, remembering to give the tray a decent shake halfway through to make sure everything is well coated.

While your sausages are cooking, bring a big pan of water to the boil. Add the squash and sweet potatoes, bring back to the boil, then turn down the heat and leave to simmer for 12 to 15 minutes, until tender. Drain in a colander and return the veg to the pan.

Add a glug of olive oil, season well with salt and pepper and mash away.

Serve a generous scoop of squash mash piled up with the sausages, apples and sticky gravy, and serve with Italian-style broccoli (page 237).

Serves 4

1 portion of your 5-a-day

8 good-quality pork sausages
2 apples, peeled, cored and
    cut into 8 wedges
2 tablespoons wholegrain
    mustard
2 tablespoons runny honey
a good splash of apple juice
1 butternut squash, peeled
    and cut into small chunks
2 sweet potatoes, peeled and
    cut into small chunks
extra virgin olive oil

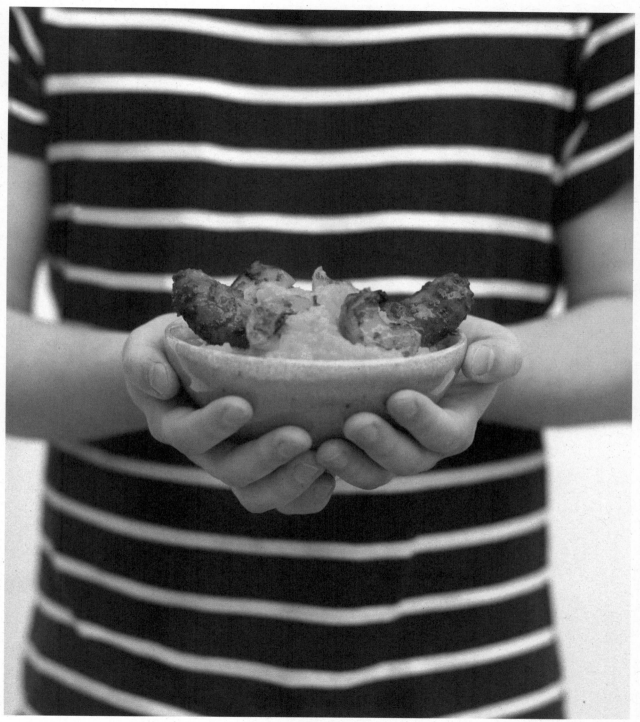

'In my hands, I hold the secret of eternal life. And some sausages.'

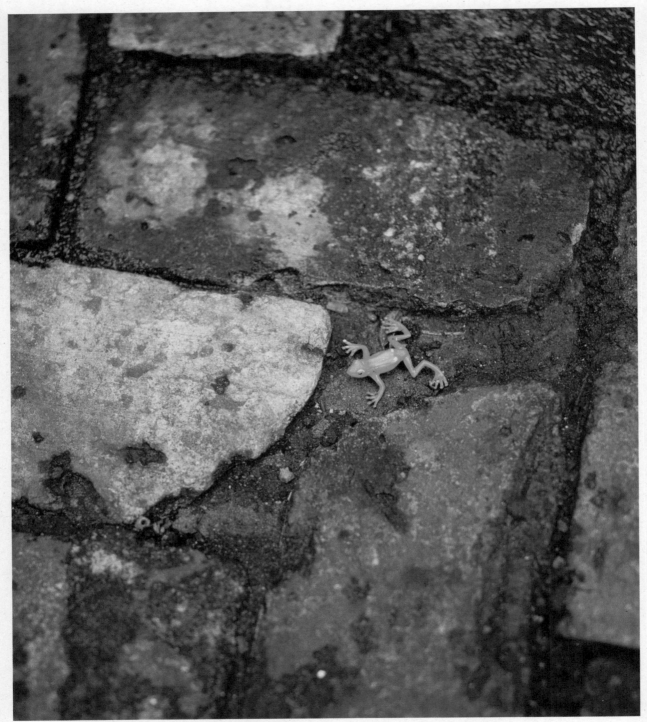

'Wish I was a chameleon.'

# Frog-in-a-ditch

**Toad-in-the-hole, sausages in batter, banging Yorkshire pudding – it tastes just as good whatever you call it.**

2 large free-range eggs
300ml milk
125g plain flour
olive oil
6 good-quality pork sausages,
   pricked all over
2 red onions, peeled and cut
   into wedges
2 sprigs of rosemary, leaves
   picked

Preheat your oven to 220°C/425°F/gas mark 7.

Whisk the eggs and milk together in a bowl, adding the flour bit by bit for a lump-free batter. Allow to stand for about 20 minutes before using.

Heat a good glug of olive oil in a big roasting tray and fry your sausages until golden on all sides. Add the onions and rosemary leaves and cook for a few more minutes. Add another glug of oil and turn up the heat until it starts to smoke. Pour in your batter and put the tray straight into the oven.

Bake for 25 to 30 minutes. Don't be tempted to open the oven or your Yorkshire pudding will deflate like a sad lilo. Check it by looking through the oven window.

After 30 minutes, or once the batter is golden brown, serve your toad-in-the-hole, frog-in-a-ditch or sausages-in-Yorkshire-pudding in big slabs, with a scoop of bright mash (page 199) and a helping of French peas (page 245) or French beans (244).

# Honey roast gammon

We left the pineapple ring out of this gammon ensemble. You can of course add a ring or two if you like. It's your tea, after all.

counts towards your 5-a-day

For the ham
- 1.5kg boneless gammon, tied up with string
- 1 big leek, washed, trimmed and roughly chopped
- 1 carrot, peeled and roughly chopped
- 1 stick of celery, roughly chopped
- 1 cinnamon stick
- 1.5 litres cloudy apple juice
- 3 tablespoons runny honey

For the sauce
- 50g salted butter
- 2 tablespoons plain flour
- 200ml milk

Put the gammon into a big pot, cover with water and bring to the boil. Lift out the gammon and pour away the water, then put the gammon back into the pan with all the other gammon ingredients apart from the honey. Top up with fresh water to completely cover the gammon and bring to the boil. Reduce the heat and simmer for 1½ hours, until cooked right through.

Preheat your oven to 200°C/400°F/gas mark 6.

Transfer the gammon and all the bits into a roasting tray. Spread the honey over the gammon and bake in the oven for 20 to 30 minutes, until it is golden and crispy. If the gammon starts to look a little dry, spoon over some of the cooking juices to keep it nice and tender.

Meanwhile, make the sauce. Melt the butter in a small saucepan, and when it is bubbling add the flour. Cook for a minute or so, then add the milk bit by bit, beating it in until it has all been added. Don't worry if your sauce goes lumpy – just cheat and sieve out any lumps.

Serve the gammon in big thick slices, drizzled with the white sauce and the appley juices, alongside a generous scoop of bright mash and lightly buttered peas.

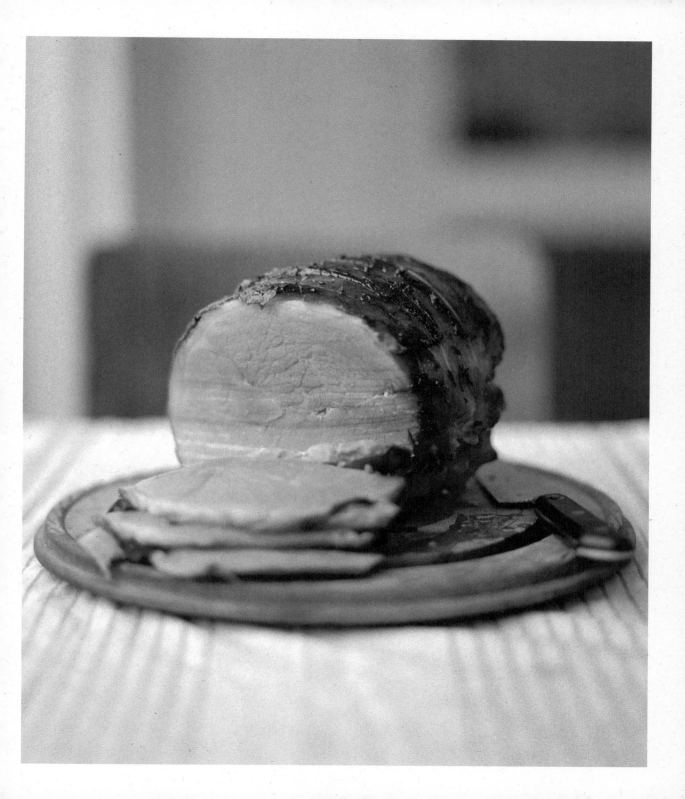

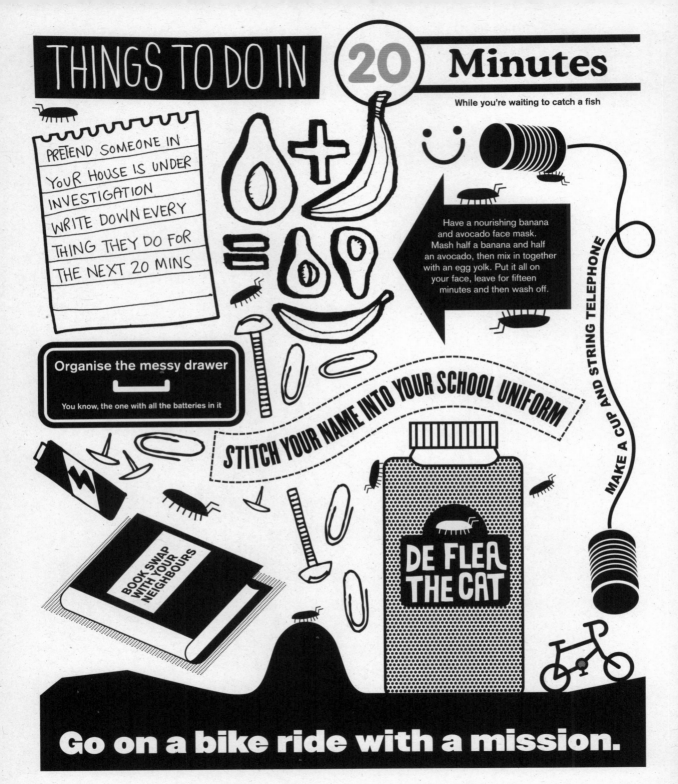

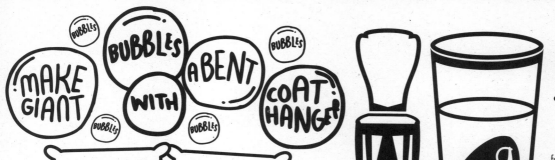

MAKE GIANT BUBBLES WITH A BENT COAT HANGER

CHANGE YOUR BED SHEETS

THE DUVET IS THE WORST BIT **DO IT FIRST.**

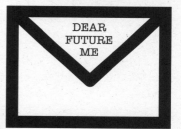

MAKE A LIVING ROOM OBSTACLE COURSE

## make a bouncy
# EGG

Take an egg (still in it's shell), then put it in a glass and cover with vinegar. Leave for a week and take it out. It will feel weird, look transparent and will bounce a bit when dropped gently (not from too high mind).

## MAKE YOUR TOP 10 LISTS

| FILMS | ALBUMS | SMELLS |
|---|---|---|
| 1. | 1. | 1. |
| 2. | 2. | 2. |
| 3. | 3. | 3. |
| 4. | 4. | 4. |
| 5. | 5. | 5. |
| 6. | 6. | 6. |
| 7. | 7. | 7. |
| 8. | 8. | 8. |
| 9. | 9. | 9. |
| 10. | 10. | 10. |

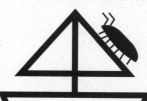

PLANT FLOWERS SEEDS HERBS

DEAR FUTURE ME

Write a letter to yourself 10 years in the future...

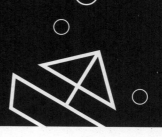

BUILD SOME BOATS OUT OF STUFF THAT'S LYING ABOUT THE HOUSE. RACE THEM IN THE BATH. FIRST TO SINK LOSES.

# Lamb kofte pittas

Pockets of spicy, lamby goodness. For a DIY dinner with a difference, pop all the kofte, salad and dressing into separate bowls and let everyone fill their own pittas. Better still, make a double batch and then freeze half for a future dinner.

Serves 4
counts towards your 5-a-day

For the koftes
1 tablespoon cumin seeds
1 tablespoon coriander seeds
olive oil
1 red onion, peeled and finely
    chopped
2 garlic cloves, peeled and
    finely chopped
1 courgette, grated
500g minced lamb
a pinch of smoked paprika
zest of 1 lemon
a few sprigs of mint, leaves
    picked and chopped

For the minty yoghurt
a few sprigs of coriander
a few sprigs of mint
juice of 1 lemon
8 tablespoons plain yoghurt

To serve
4 wooden skewers, soaked in
    cold water
4 wholemeal pittas or
    flatbread

Preheat your oven to 150°C/300°F/gas mark 2.

Toast the cumin and coriander seeds in a dry frying pan over a medium heat, then give them a bash in a pestle and mortar.

Add a drizzle of olive oil to the pan and fry the onion and garlic for 5 minutes over a medium heat. Add the grated courgette and cook for about 10 minutes, until soft.

Transfer the mixture to a bowl and set aside. When cool, add the minced lamb, bashed spices and paprika. Add the lemon zest and chopped mint, season with salt and pepper and mix together with your hands.

Divide the lamb mixture into 4, then form into sausage shapes and poke a skewer into the end of each one. If you don't have any skewers, flatten the mixture into patties instead.

Pop the flatbreads into the oven to warm up. Heat a drizzle of olive oil in a griddle or frying pan until slightly smoking and cook the koftes for about 10 minutes, turning every couple of minutes.

To make the minty yoghurt, put the coriander, mint, lemon juice and yoghurt into a bowl. Add a little olive oil, season with salt and pepper and mix well.

Serve your koftes inside the warm flatbreads, drizzled with the minty yoghurt and topped with chop chop salad (page 220).

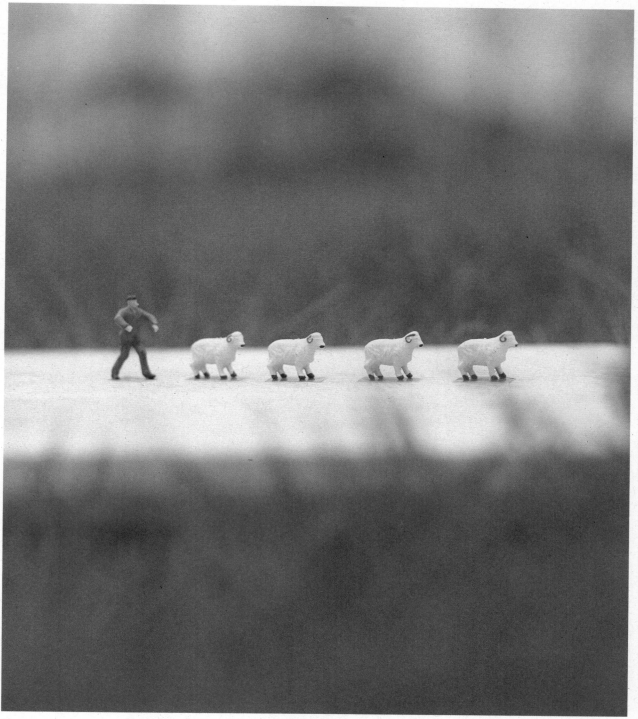

The sheepdog trials were going rather well, considering there was no sheepdog.

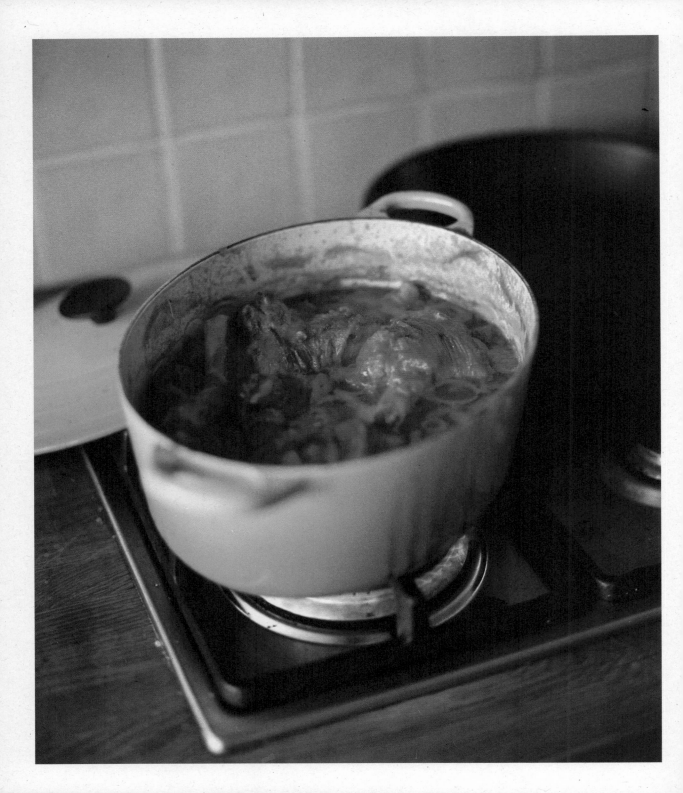

# Lamb shank tagine

A tagine is a special Moroccan cooking pot with a funny conical lid. But you can still make a fine tagine without the requisite pointy cover. Leave it to bubble away while you get on with something else. It'll taste all the better for not being rushed.

Serves 4
2 portions of your 5-a-day

For the tagine
olive oil
4 garlic cloves, peeled and
    finely sliced
2 red onions, peeled and
    finely sliced
1 teaspoon ground cinnamon
1 teaspoon smoked paprika
1 teaspoon cumin seeds
1 teaspoon coriander seeds
2 x 400g tins of chopped
    tomatoes
½ a medium butternut squash,
    peeled and cut into 3cm
    chunks
a small handful of dried
    apricots, roughly chopped
500ml chicken or vegetable
    stock
1 lemon
a pinch of saffron strands
4 lamb shanks

To serve
4 flatbreads
400g steamed couscous
4 tablespoons plain yoghurt
a big bunch of coriander

Preheat your oven to 180°C/350°F/gas mark 4.

Heat a drizzle of olive oil in your casserole and cook the garlic and onions over a medium heat for about 10 minutes, until soft. Add the spices and fry for another minute.

Next add the tomatoes, squash, apricots and stock.

Use a potato peeler to peel a few strips off the lemon and add these to the pan, along with the saffron strands.

Season the lamb shanks with salt and pepper and add to the pan, making sure they are covered by the liquid. Then put the lid on and put the casserole into the oven for 2 hours, until the sauce is lovely and thick and the meat is melting away from the bone.

If the sauce needs thickening, just put the pan on to the hob for a few minutes to reduce it down.

About 10 minutes before serving, pop the flatbreads into the oven and make up your couscous according to the instructions on the packet.

Serve each lamb shank with a helping of green salad (page 211), a warm flatbread, a scoop of couscous and a dollop of yoghurt, topped with roughly chopped fresh coriander.

# Slow-cooked beef stew

Sometimes, slow can be good. Getting into a hot bath, for example. Driving on icy roads. Being stuck in traffic when you're sat next to someone attractive on the bus. All this stuff is better for being that bit slower. Same with this recipe. Pop it on to cook and then put your feet up, safe in the knowledge that dinner is quietly bubbling away. Slowly.

Preheat your oven to 180°C/350°F/gas mark 4.

Find a big casserole with a lid and put it on a medium heat. Season the beef with salt and pepper. Add some butter to the casserole and fry the meat until well browned. Then tip the beef on to a plate and place the casserole back on the heat.

Add the onions and carrots and cook until soft, then add the butternut squash, beef and flour and cook for a couple of minutes, until the flour has turned pale brown.

Add the bay leaves, thyme, tomatoes and balsamic vinegar. Crumble in the stock cube and chuck in 2 mugfuls (around 400ml) of water.

Put the lid on and pop the casserole into the oven for 1 to 1½ hours, until the beef is tender and the sauce has thickened nicely. If you want your sauce that bit thicker, just put it on the hob over a high heat for 5 minutes to reduce down.

Serve with a big scoop of bright mash (page 199) and some simple spinach (page 226).

Serves 4
2 portions of your 5-a-day

500g stewing beef, cut into bite-sized chunks
a knob of butter
2 red onions, peeled and roughly chopped
2 carrots, peeled and roughly chopped
½ a butternut squash, cut into big chunks
1 tablespoon plain flour
2 bay leaves
a few sprigs of thyme
1 x 400g tin of chopped tomatoes
3 tablespoons balsamic vinegar
1 beef stock cube

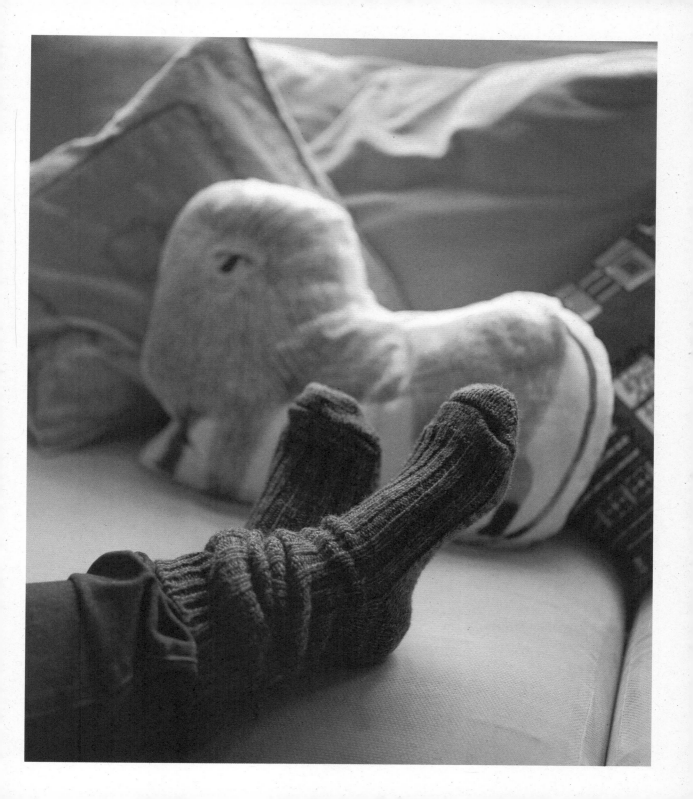

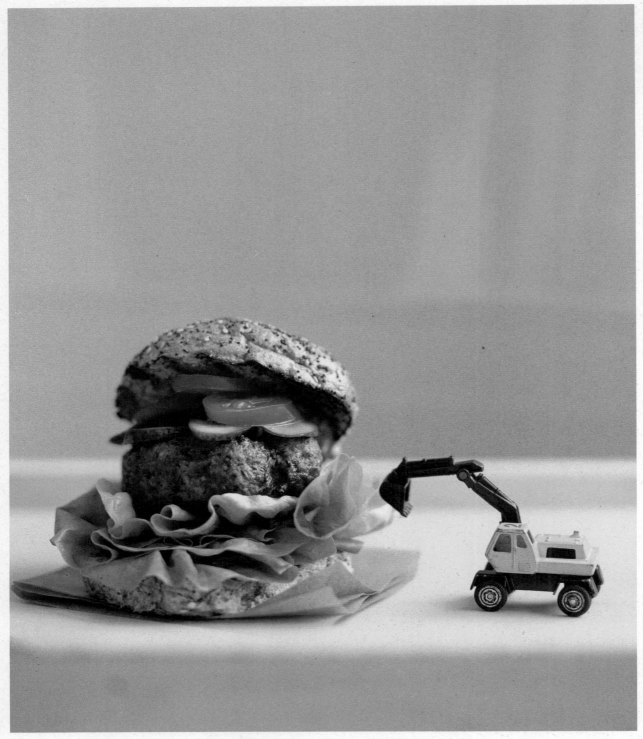

'We've got a big one here, Gavin.'

# Build-your-own burgers

You grows them, you knows them. Or in the case of these homemade burgers, you get everyone to build their own to guarantee dinner being eaten. Not as catchy but the same principles apply.

Serves 4

1 portion of your 5-a-day

For the burgers

a little drizzle of olive oil

1 red onion, peeled and finely chopped

2 garlic cloves, peeled and finely chopped

1 teaspoon English mustard

50g Cheddar cheese, grated

a small bunch of parsley, finely chopped

2 handfuls of breadcrumbs

1 free-range egg

500g lean minced beef

4 of your favourite bread rolls

For the topping

3 tomatoes, sliced

a handful of round lettuce leaves

a handful of gherkins, chopped

Heat a pan over a medium heat, add a splash of olive oil and cook the onion and garlic for about 10 minutes, until soft.

Put the onion and garlic mix into a big bowl and leave to cool. Beat the egg and then add it along with the mustard, cheese, chopped parsley, breadcrumbs, egg and minced beef to the onion and garlic. Use your hands to mix it all together, then divide the mixture into 4 and get everyone to shape their burgers.

Before you start shaping, wash your hands and then wet them in cold water to stop the mix sticking to your fingers. Take a blob of burger mix in your hands and shape and mould it round and round into a burger shape. Then flatten it out to about 1.5cm thick – it'll shrink a bit during cooking.

Once shaped and flattened, pop your burgers into the fridge for at least half an hour to firm up.

Heat a dry frying pan or griddle pan until it's nice and hot. Cook the burgers for 4 minutes or so on each side, until they are cooked through, and pop them on to a plate covered with foil to keep them warm till they are all ready.

Wipe out the pan, pop it back on the heat and toast your buns. Then put your toppings onto plates and lay them all out on the table.

Let everyone build their own burgers and serve with rainbow chips (page 224) and chop chop salad (page 220).

# Failsafe spag bol

**Life's like spaghetti. It should be nice and long but sometimes it sticks to the pan. So you know what to do: just buy a non-stick pan.**

Serves 4

1½ portions of your 5-a-day

olive oil

a knob of butter

1 onion, peeled and finely chopped

2 carrots, peeled and finely chopped

1 stick of celery, finely chopped

4 rashers of smoked bacon or pancetta, roughly chopped

500g minced beef

1 big glass of white wine

200ml milk

a pinch of grated nutmeg

2 x 400g tins of chopped tomatoes

400g dried spaghetti

some Parmesan cheese, for grating

Heat a splash of olive oil and a knob of butter in a large casserole, then add the onion and cook slowly for 10 minutes, until soft. Add the carrots, celery and bacon and cook for a further 5 minutes.

Add the minced beef, season with salt and pepper, and fry until the mince starts to brown. Pour in the wine and simmer over a medium heat until it has completely evaporated, then add the milk and do the same.

Once all the milk has gone, grate in some nutmeg and add the tinned tomatoes. Turn down the heat and allow to simmer, uncovered, for 1½ to 3 hours, depending on how much time you have. The longer you can leave it, the better. Give it the occasional stir and top up with water if needed.

After 1½ hours, or however long you've left it, bring a big pan of water to the boil. Add a pinch of salt, and once the water is boiling, cook the spaghetti for about 8 minutes, until al dente.

Once the pasta is cooked, dip a mug into the pan and fill with the pasta water. Set aside. Drain the spaghetti, add to the bolognese sauce and stir it all together. If it looks a little dry, add in some water from your mug. Serve your spag bol in big scoops topped with a sprinkling of grated Parmesan.

The cooked sauce will keep well in the fridge for a few days and can easily be frozen once cooled (some would argue that it tastes better the day after).

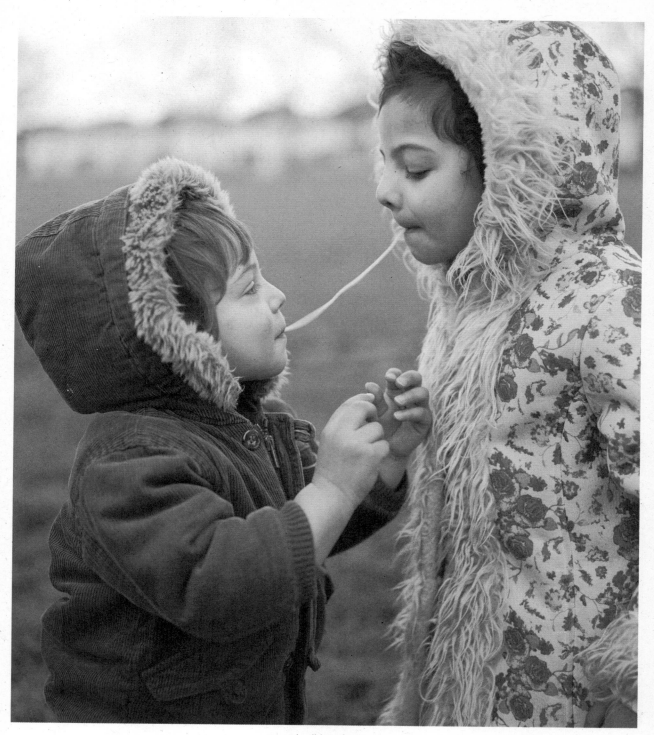

Who'll bite first?

# Sticky barbecue ribs

When it comes to ribs, the stickier the better. But things sure can get messy, so if you're having people round for supper, put a scattering of rose petals in a few bowls of warm water and pop them on the table. However, if you're eating this in your tracksuit, then flat-pack finger bowls (a.k.a. the wet wipe) are fine.

**Serves 4**

**counts towards your 5-a-day**

4 half racks of baby back ribs
1 red onion, peeled and finely chopped
4 garlic cloves, peeled and finely chopped
olive oil
1 teaspoon cumin seeds
1 teaspoon fennel seeds
a few sprigs of thyme, stalks removed
1 tablespoon smoked paprika
grated zest and juice of 1 orange
150ml cloudy apple juice or water
150ml tomato or traffic-light ketchup (for a recipe see page 310)
2 tablespoons runny honey
1 tablespoon balsamic vinegar

Either blitz the onion and garlic in a food processor or chop them very finely by hand, then cook them in a medium pan with a good glug of olive oil for about 5 minutes, or until soft.

Bash the cumin and fennel seeds in a pestle and mortar and add to the pan. Cook for another couple of minutes, then add the rest of the ingredients (apart from the ribs), bring to the boil, then reduce the heat and leave to simmer for 10 minutes.

Once cooled, put the sauce through a sieve, using a metal spoon to smooth any onions through.

Preheat your oven to 180°C/350°F/gas mark 4. Put the ribs into a big roasting tray.

Rub the ribs with half the cooled barbecue sauce. Add a splash of water to the tray and cover with foil.

Cook in the oven for 40 minutes, then remove the foil, brush over a bit more barbecue sauce and cook for another 15 minutes, until the ribs are sticky.

Serve with chop chop salad (page 220), smoky potato wedges (page 202) and several fingerbowls.

# Cottage pie

Serves 4

2 portions of your 5-a-day

## For the pie bit

olive oil

1 big leek, washed, trimmed and finely sliced

2 garlic cloves, peeled and finely sliced

2 carrots, peeled and roughly chopped

1 stick of celery, roughly chopped

1 parsnip, peeled and roughly chopped

500g minced beef

1 teaspoon smoked paprika

a splash of Worcestershire sauce

a few sprigs of thyme

1 x 400g tin of chopped tomatoes

1 chicken or vegetable stock cube

## For the cottage bit

2 carrots, peeled and cut into small chunks

1 sweet potato, peeled and cut into small chunks

2 large potatoes, peeled and cut into small chunks

a couple of knobs of butter

freshly grated nutmeg

a splash of milk

A quick lesson in pies: Shepherd's = lamb. Cottage = beef. Lentils = Sussex/hippy. If you fancy a meat-free pie, use the same quantity of lentils. No need to fry them off first. Just add them in with the rest of the veg.

Preheat your oven to 180°C/350°F/gas mark 4.

Get a good sized frying pan on a medium heat, add a splash of olive oil and cook the leek, garlic, carrots, celery and parsnip for about 10 minutes, until soft.

Turn up the heat and stir in the minced beef. Fry for a few minutes, until all the meat has changed from pink to brown, then add the smoked paprika, Worcestershire sauce and thyme leaves. Fry for another minute or so, then add the tomatoes, stock cube and a mugful (about 200ml) of water.

Turn down the heat and leave to simmer for 30 minutes or so, stirring occasionally and adding a splash of water if it starts to stick.

While the mince is cooking, make the topping. Put your carrots, sweet potato and potatoes into a pan and cover with boiling water. Add a pinch of salt, then bring to the boil and cook for 12 to15 minutes, until soft.

Drain the veg, tip back into the pan and mash them, adding a couple of knobs of butter, a good grating of nutmeg and a splash of milk.

Tip your pie mixture into a big pie dish, top with the mash and use a spoon to spread it out evenly. Rake it over with a fork and bake in the oven for 40 minutes, until golden and bubbling.

Serve with peas or steamed broccoli.

# Chicken, bacon and leek pie

For the flakiest, crispiest pastry in the world: keep it cold and handle as little as possible. For the flakiest, crumbliest milk chocolate in the land: yellow wrapper, third shelf down, next to the Yorkies.

Preheat your oven to 190°C/375°F/gas mark 5.

Heat a little olive oil in a frying pan and fry the leeks and garlic over a medium heat for 10 to 15 minutes, until the leeks are soft. Remove them from the pan and set aside, then put the pan back on the heat.

Add some more oil to the pan and add the chicken and bacon. Cook until the chicken starts to brown, then add the leeks, squash, thyme and flour and stir for a few more minutes. Then add the stock and simmer for 10 minutes.

Meanwhile, dust a clean work surface with flour and roll out the pastry, using a rolling pin, to about 5mm thickness and big enough to fit over your pie dish. Beat the egg and milk together and place to one side. Tip the chicken filling into the pie dish and brush the edge of the dish with the egg mixture. Then roll the pastry around the rolling pin and drape it over the top.

Use a fork to press the edges of the pastry to the side of the dish, then trim off any excess and brush the top of your pie with the egg mixture. Make a little hole in the middle to allow some air to escape, and use any leftover pastry to decorate the top with leaves, shapes or the names of all the pie eaters, remembering to brush any decorations with egg mix (see pages 136 to 137 for ideas).

Bake in the oven for about 45 to 50 minutes, until the pastry is golden brown. To balance out this treat of a tea, serve with a big scoop of bright mash (page 199) and some steamed broccoli.

You can also make the pie up to the stage just before you brush with egg, then allow to cool completely and freeze – it will keep for a few months.

Serves 4
counts towards your 5-a-day

olive oil
2 leeks, trimmed, washed and roughly chopped
2 garlic cloves, peeled and roughly chopped
8 chicken thighs, skinned, boned and cut into bite-sized pieces
4 rashers of smoked streaky bacon, roughly chopped
½ a small butternut squash, deseeded, peeled and cut into small chunks
a few sprigs of thyme
2 tablespoons plain flour
200ml chicken stock
1 x 500g packet of puff pastry
1 large free-range egg
a splash of milk

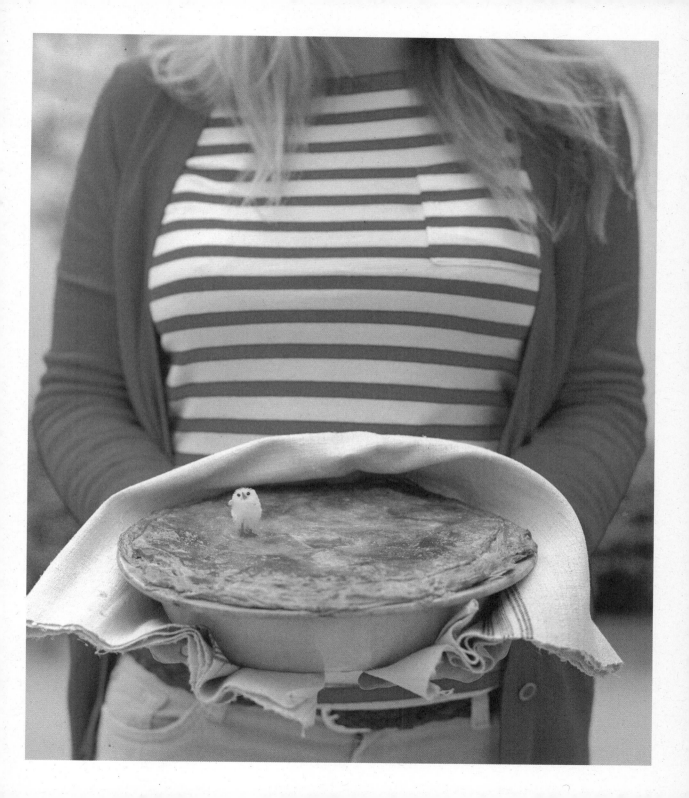

# Proper chicken nuggets

**These work just as well with white fish, like pollack or coley. Just make sure your fish is well boned beforehand.**

### Serves 4
100g polenta

4 cream crackers or oatcakes

zest of 1 lemon

a few sprigs of parsley, finely chopped

2 tablespoons plain flour

2 large free-range eggs, beaten

4 free-range chicken breasts, sliced into long strips

Preheat your oven to 180°C/350°F/gas mark 4.

Put the polenta, crackers or oatcakes, lemon zest and parsley into a food processor and whizz to fine breadcrumbs. If you don't have a food processor, put the whole lot into a sandwich bag and bash with a rolling pin instead.

Put the breadcrumbs on one plate and the flour on another. Beat the eggs in a bowl.

Dip the chicken strips one by one first into the flour, then into the egg, then into the breadcrumbs and place on a lightly greased baking tray.

Bake in the oven for 15 to 20 minutes, until the chicken is cooked through and the breadcrumb coating is golden.

Serve with smoky potato wedges (page 202) and chop chop salad (page 220) or homemade beans (page 71).

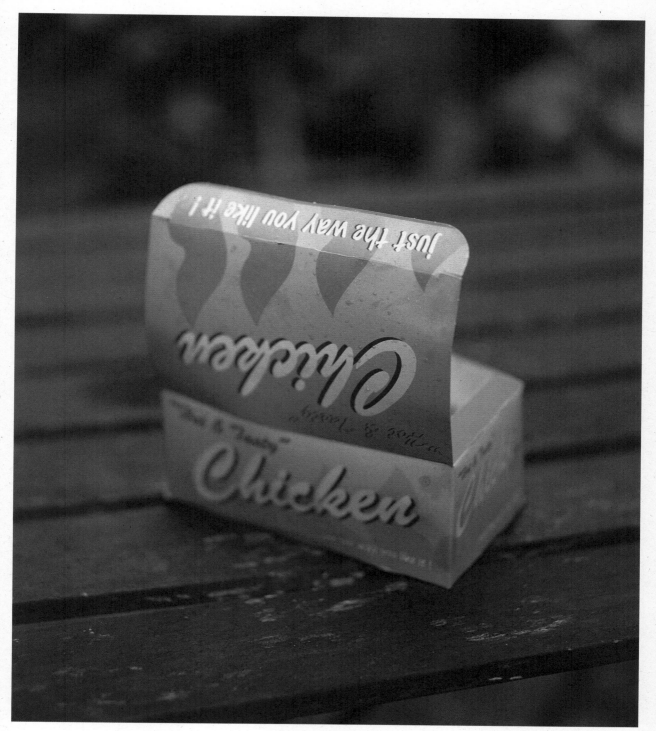

Serving suggestion

# Mexican chicken fajitas

2½ portions of your 5-a-day

## For the chicken

4 free-range chicken breasts

zest of 1 lime

1 teaspoon smoked paprika

1 teaspoon ground cumin

olive oil

2 red peppers, deseeded and
cut into thin strips

1 red onion, peeled and cut
into thin strips

## For the salsa

a big handful of cherry
tomatoes, quartered

1 spring onion, finely sliced

½ a red chilli, deseeded and
finely chopped

a few sprigs of coriander,
roughly chopped

a splash of extra virgin olive oil

a splash of balsamic vinegar

## For the guacamole

2 ripe avocados

juice of 1 lime

## To serve

8 wholemeal flour tortillas

a tub of soured cream or
crème fraîche

100g Cheddar or Manchego
cheese, grated

You can also make these using an equivalent amount of steak. For a veggie option, griddled sweet potato or butternut squash (parboiled before griddling) works really well, as do the homemade beans (page 71). Wrap away.

Preheat your oven to 150°C/300°F/gas mark 2.

Slice each chicken breast into 6 thin strips and pop them into a bowl. Add the lime zest, paprika, cumin, salt, pepper and a splash of olive oil. Stir until the chicken is thoroughly coated, then set aside.

To make sure your griddle pan is really hot, put it on a medium heat while you make the salsa and guacamole.

Pop all the salsa ingredients into a food processor and pulse till chunky. Or if you don't have a food processor, finely chop all the ingredients and put into a serving bowl.

Cut the avocados in half and remove the stones, then scoop the flesh into a bowl and mash with the lime juice. Season well with salt and pepper and put into another serving bowl. Then wrap the tortillas in foil and pop into the oven to warm through.

Your griddle pan should be really hot by now, so cook the peppers and onion until charred or soft (depending on which you prefer). Put them on to a plate and place in the oven to keep warm.

Next, griddle the chicken for 8 minutes, until blackened on the outside, and put it into a serving bowl.

Take the tortillas and vegetables out of the oven and place them on the table with the chicken, salsa, guacamole, soured cream or crème fraîche and grated cheese. Get everyone to make their own fajitas and serve with chop chop salad (page 220).

# Classy lemony chicken

This is not the dish you get in Chinese restaurants that arrives on the spinny table with some yellow gravy. This lemony chicken is a simple take on the French classic. You can serve it on a Lazy Susan if you have one. But it's probably easier to use a plate.

Serves 4
counts towards your 5-a-day

olive oil
2 leeks, trimmed, washed and
    roughly chopped
2 garlic cloves, peeled and
    chopped
a small bunch of thyme
1 glass of white wine
about 400ml good chicken
    stock
2 lemons
8 free-range boneless chicken
    thighs, skin on
a bunch of parsley, dill or
    tarragon, or a mixture,
    chopped

Preheat your oven to 150°C/300°F/gas mark 2.

Get yourself a large casserole and add a good splash of olive oil. Add the leeks, garlic and thyme and cook on a low heat – you don't want the veg to brown at all – for about 10 to 15 minutes, to bring out their sweetness.

When the leeks are soft and sweet, add the wine, stock and the zest and juice of both lemons. Leave to simmer for about 30 minutes.

Season the chicken with salt and pepper if you like and put it into the casserole skin side down. Let it sizzle away until the chicken is deeply golden on all sides.

Take the chicken out of the pan, put it on a plate and pop it in the oven to keep warm.

Remove the thyme sprigs and serve the chicken with the sauce poured over and the chopped herbs sprinkled on top. This goes nicely with some simple boiled potatoes or steamed rice and French beans (page 244).

# The best roast chicken and stuffing ever

Serves 6
1½ portions of your 5-a-day

**For the roast chicken**
1 free-range chicken,
   weighing around 1.6kg
2 red onions, peeled and cut
   into wedges
2 carrots, peeled and cut into
   chunks
2 sticks of celery, cut into
   chunks
3 garlic cloves, unpeeled
1 lemon
a small bunch of thyme
a few bay leaves

**For the stuffing**
6 rashers of smoked streaky
   bacon, chopped
2 red onions, peeled and
   finely chopped
1 stick of celery, finely
   chopped
a few sprigs of thyme
a handful of dried apricots,
   chopped
1 apple, cored and finely
   diced
1 orange
6 good-quality sausages
2 handfuls of brown
   breadcrumbs
1 large free-range egg,
   beaten

There's nothing in all the land quite like a roast chicken. Especially when you follow it with an afternoon of big newspapers, old Bond films on the telly and snoozing. Here's our favourite way to make it – just don't forget the gravy (page 193).

Preheat your oven to 200°C/400°F/gas mark 6 and take your chicken out of the fridge so it's not too cold when it goes in the oven.

First, make the stuffing. Put the bacon into a frying pan and cook until it starts to brown, then add the onions and celery and cook for 10 minutes over a low heat, until soft. Strip the thyme leaves from the stalks, add and cook for another minute or so.

Take off the heat, and stir in the apricots and apple. Finely grate in the zest of the orange. Next, squeeze the sausagemeat out of their skins and add to the mixture, then add the breadcrumbs and beaten egg and give everything a really good mix. Roll the stuffing into ping-pong-size balls and put them on a roasting tray.

Back to the chicken. Put all the veg into a large roasting tray and add the unpeeled garlic cloves. Place your chicken on top and season it well on all sides. Cut the lemon in half and stuff it inside the chicken, along with the thyme and bay leaves. Roast for 45 minutes, then put the tray of stuffing balls into the oven and roast for another 45 minutes.

After the chicken has been in the oven for about 1½ hours, it should be perfectly cooked. Check by sticking a fork into one of the legs. If it's cooked, the juices should run clear.

Remove the roasting tray from the oven. Leaving the vegetables in the tray, transfer the chicken on to a plate or wooden chopping board and cover with kitchen foil. Then make the gravy (page 193).

Serve your roast chicken with the gravy, stuffing balls, crunchy lemon roast potatoes (page 202) and Italian style broccoli (page 237).

# TIMINGS

10AM        OVEN ON

            MAKE STUFFING
11:00       PREP CHICKEN

            CHICKEN INTO OVEN
11:45       PREP VEG (BROC/CARR/PARS/SPUD)

            STUFFING INTO OVEN
12:00       PARBOIL SPUDS & PARSNIPS

            SPUDS & PARSNIPS INTO OVEN
            LAY TABLE
12:15       WASH UP DIRTY STUFF

12:30       GIVE SPUDS A SHAKE

            TAKE CHICKEN OUT → FOIL
12:45       STEAM VEG

1pm    SERVE    STUFFING, SPUDS + PARSNIPS OUT

# Roast duck with spuds and plums

If only we could magic the wonder that is roast duck into a smoothie, then we'd be feasting on it morning, noon and every tea break with the crossword and possibly a chocolate digestive. Till that special day arrives, here's our favourite recipe instead.

Serves 4–6
1 portion of your 5-a-day

For the roast duck
1 large duck (about 1.5kg)
1 large orange, cut in half
3 sprigs of rosemary
4 bay leaves
a small knob of fresh ginger, peeled and thinly sliced
1kg new potatoes
10 red plums, halved and quartered
1 whole garlic bulb, unpeeled

For the gravy (see page 193)
1 tablespoon plain flour
a generous splash of booze (red wine or Marsala work really well)
200ml hot chicken or vegetable stock
2 tablespoons damson/blackberry/blackcurrant jam

Preheat your oven to 180°C/350°F/gas mark 4.

Place the duck in a large roasting tray. Season well with sea salt and cracked black pepper and rub into the skin thoroughly. Stuff the orange halves, 1 rosemary sprig, 2 bay leaves and the sliced ginger inside the duck and roast in the oven for about 2 hours. Drain the fat from the tray into a bowl every 30 minutes and keep for later.

While the duck is cooking, bring a pan of water to the boil and add the potatoes. Bring back to the boil, then cook them for about 5 minutes. Drain them and put them into a second roasting tray with the plums and the other 2 bay leaves. Strip the needles off the remaining rosemary sprigs and add them to the tray. Then smash the bulb of garlic into cloves and add these too. No need to peel them.

After the duck has been roasting for about 45 minutes, pour the fat you've collected over the potatoes and pop them into the oven. Keep draining the fat off the duck as it cooks, for the gravy.

After 1¼ hours, check the duck is cooked by sticking a metal skewer into one of the legs. The juices should run clear if it's ready. If not, pop it back into the oven for a few more minutes.

Once cooked, take out the garlic cloves, remove the duck from the tray and pop it on to a plate. Then cover with foil and set aside to rest. Turn the oven down to 150°C/300°F/gas mark 2 and pop the potatoes back in to keep warm.

Drain any remaining fat from the duck tray and make the gravy (page 193). Serve the roast duck shredded and piled on top of the potatoes and plums, with steamed broccoli and a drizzle of gravy.

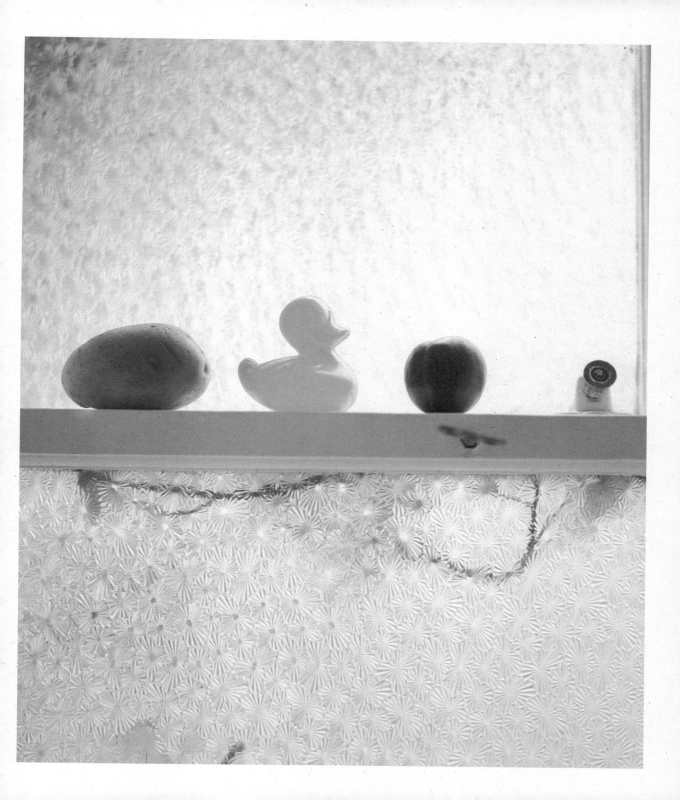

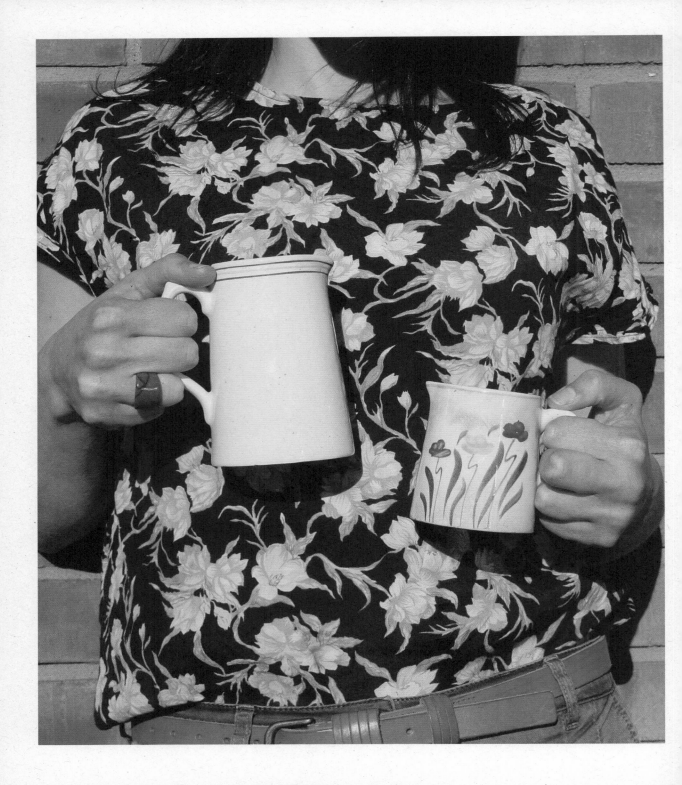

# Don't forget the gravy

**After all, it's the only reason you ever make a roast dinner (if we're being completely honest).**

## Roast chicken gravy

2 tablespoons plain flour

500ml scrumpy cider or apple juice

Finally, make the gravy. Place the roasting tin on a high heat, spooning off anything that looks oily. Get the whole lot heated up, then use a potato masher to mash all the veg that you cooked with the chicken to a pulp, remembering to squeeze the roasted garlic out of its skins.

Add a couple of tablespoons of flour and stir for a minute or so, until the flour is starting to brown. Pour in the cider or apple juice and simmer for 5 to 10 minutes, until the gravy is as thick as you want it to be, then pour it into a jug.

## Roast duck gravy

leftover duck fat

1 tablespoon plain flour

a generous splash of booze (red wine or Marsala work really well)

200ml hot chicken or vegetable stock

2 tablespoons damson/ blackberry/blackcurrant jam

Pour the duck fat into a roasting tray and place over a medium heat. Add the flour and use a metal spoon to stir into the fat for a couple of minutes, until it starts to brown.

Add the wine and keep stirring for another minute, then add the stock bit by bit, until the gravy is as thick as you like it. Finally, stir in the jam and pour the gravy into a serving jug.

# GOOD THINGS TO HAVE FOR

---

# SIDES

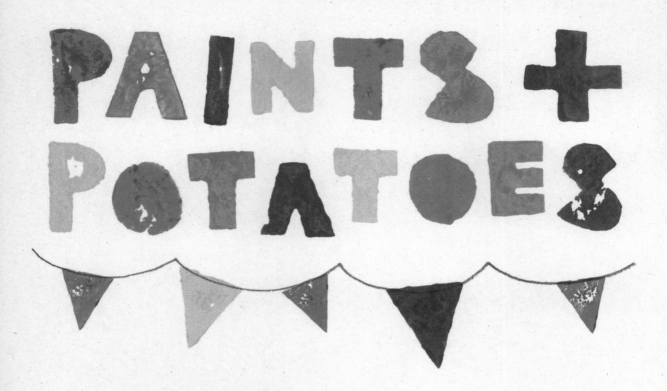

# PAINTS + POTATOES

One potato, two potato, three potato, four. Here's our easy four step guide to creating the perfect potato printed picture.

Before you get started, make sure you've got your potato print kit sorted.

## You will need:

Potatoes big enough for cutting into, some paper or card for printing on, a kitchen knife (for grown ups only), water-based paints, a saucer, some felt tip pens, some kitchen roll, a big table with some newspaper laid out and an old t-shirt to wear (things could get a bit messy).

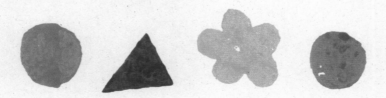

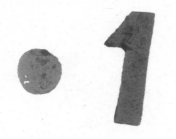

Sketch out the shapes you'd like to print onto some paper. Simple is best. So think circles, squares and triangles rather than dodecahedrons and outlines of countries.

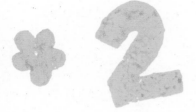

Ask a grown up to cut your potato in half and then use a sharp pencil to mark out your shape onto the flat side of your spud. Then get a grown up to cut away the bits round your shape so it sticks out. Repeat for all the other shapes you want to print. **Tip:** if you're printing letters or numbers, make sure you do them back to front.

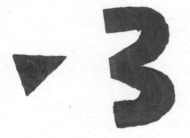

Next, pour your paint into a saucer, dip your potato shapes into the paint and have a quick practice on some scrap paper. Then print away. To print a different colour, give your potato a wash under the cold tap. **Tip:** don't overload your spud with paint or it'll make a big splodge on your paper. Print onto scrap paper first or use a paint brush to make sure you get a nice even spread of paint.

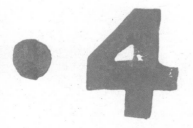

Leave your print to dry completely. Add any finishing touches with felt tip pens, coloured pencils or some glitter. Then stick on the fridge, stand back and admire your potato masterpiece. Chin stroking optional. **Tip:** adding the little details to your design is much simpler when it's dry. It's much easier to print a circle and then draw on a face than spend ages trying to cut out some eyes, a nose and a mouth.

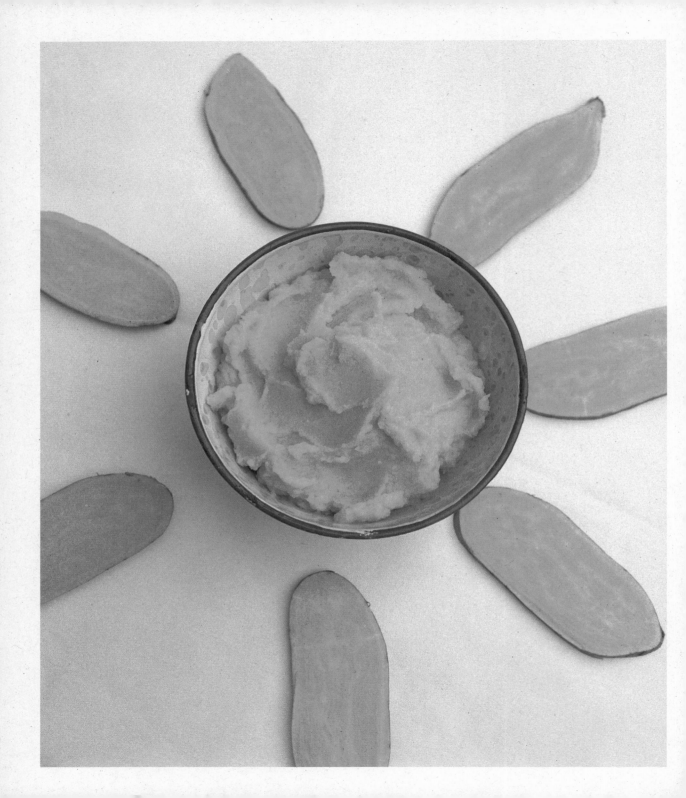

# Bright mash

**Like normal mash. Only more cheerful.**

Serves 4
1 portion of your 5-a-day

400g Desiree or other good
mashing potatoes
400g sweet potatoes
2 carrots
a big knob of butter

Peel and chop the potatoes, sweet potatoes and carrots. Bring a large pan of water to the boil and add the veg. Bring back to the boil and cook for 10 to 15 minutes, until tender.

Drain in a colander, allow to steam for a couple of minutes, then pop the veg back into the pan and mash with the butter.

Season well and serve in jolly scoops.

## Good stuff to add:

Before mashing
Add 2 big handfuls of frozen peas or sweetcorn for the last few minutes of cooking.
Add 2 tablespoons of pesto when you start the mashing.

After mashing
Stir in 2 tablespoons of roughly chopped roasted red peppers from a jar.

# Sweet potato gratin

Like what you get in fancy French restaurants. If fancy French restaurants served sweet potatoes. And paid your dad to serve dinner in his tux. (This recipe is a bit of a treat, so one for every now and then, as opposed to every night of the week.)

Serves 4
1 portion of your 5-a-day

800g sweet potatoes
2 garlic cloves, peeled and finely chopped
a few sprigs of rosemary, stalks removed
1 red chilli, deseeded and finely chopped
olive oil
250ml single cream
100g freshly grated Parmesan cheese

Preheat your oven to 180°C/350°F/gas mark 4.

Scrub the sweet potatoes and slice them as thinly as you can. Pop them into a bowl with the garlic, rosemary leaves and chopped chilli and season well with salt and pepper. Drizzle with olive oil and toss together till all the slices are well coated, then layer them in an ovenproof casserole dish.

Pour over the cream, sprinkle with the cheese and bake in the oven for 40 minutes, until golden.

# Mini potatoes in their jackets

The crunchier, the better. Leave the skins on and let your oven work its magic. Spud-in-suits never tasted so good.

Serves 6
800g new potatoes, scrubbed
olive oil

Preheat your oven to 180°C/350°F/gas mark 4.

Pop the potatoes into a baking tray and drizzle them with olive oil. Season with salt and pepper and toss the spuds until thoroughly coated.

Bake in the oven for 40 minutes, until the jackets are golden brown and crispy.

Once cooked, allow the potatoes to cool a little, then cut them open and fill them with a blob of crème fraîche, a sprinkling of grated cheese or whatever else you fancy.

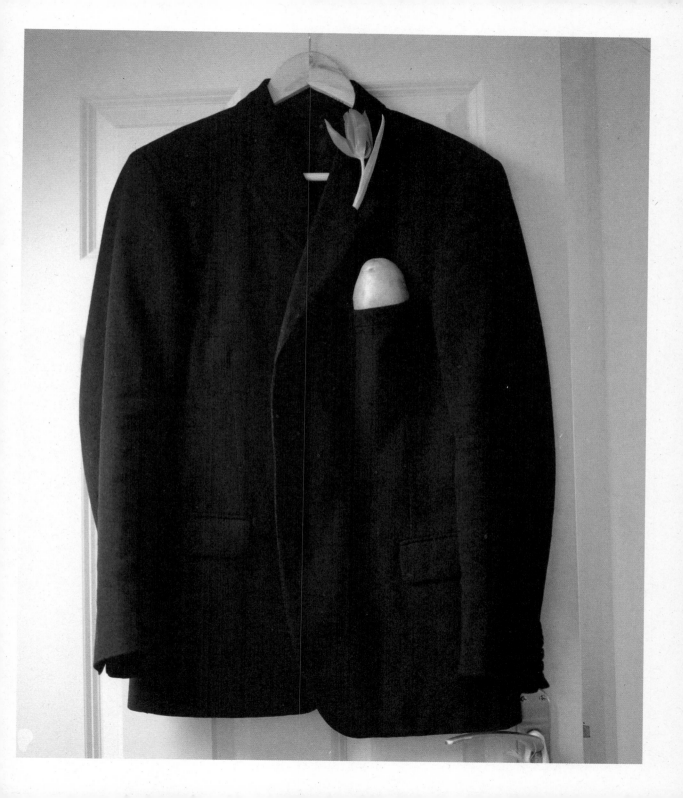

# Crunchy lemon roast potatoes

A zesty twist on the humble roast potato.

Preheat your oven to 200°C/400°F/gas mark 6.

Peel the potatoes and cut them into quarters. Put them into a big pan, cover them with boiling water from the kettle and add a pinch of salt. Bring back to the boil, then cook for 8 to 10 minutes, until the potatoes are soft around the edges. Drain them in a colander.

Put the potatoes into a roasting tray, giving them a good jiggle around so that the edges scuff up and go fluffy.

Sprinkle them with the lemon zest, then add the thyme and a generous drizzle of olive oil and season well. Give everything a good shake and roast in the oven for 40 minutes, until the potatoes are golden, remembering to give them another stir and shake halfway through.

**Serves 6**
800g King Edward or Maris
 Piper potatoes
finely grated zest of 1 lemon
a few sprigs of thyme
olive oil

# Smoky potato wedges

**Lost in the desert with only a pocketful of spices, a box of matches and a couple of spuds? Pass the time by making these wedges while you wait for the chap in the feathery headband to get the smoke rings going.**

Preheat your oven to 200°C/400°F/gas mark 6.

Bring a large pan of water to the boil. Add the potatoes and sweet potatoes, bring back to the boil, and cook for 6 to 8 minutes. Drain in a colander and set aside to dry off. Give the cumin seeds a good bash in a pestle and mortar while you're waiting.

Next, put the wedges in to a roasting tray, drizzle them with olive oil and toss with the cumin seeds and smoked paprika. Spread the wedges out and bake for 40 minutes (giving the tray a shake halfway through) until golden and crispy. Serve with traffic light ketchup (page 310).

**Serves 4**
2 large potatoes (Maris Piper
 or King Edward), scrubbed
 and cut into wedges
2 large sweet potatoes,
 scrubbed and cut into
 wedges
a pinch of cumin seeds
olive oil
1 teaspoon smoked paprika

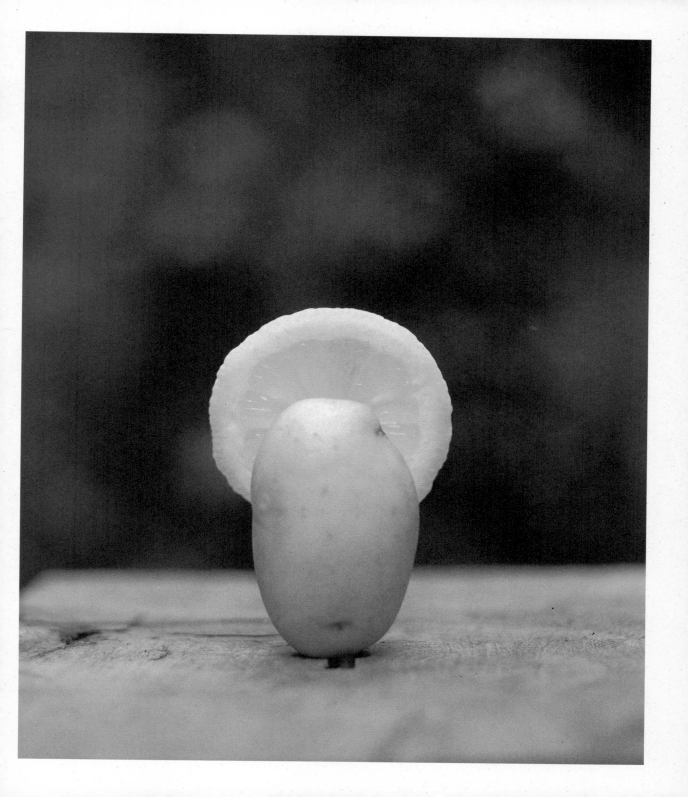

# Potato and apple rösti

We were going to call these potato and apple nests. But rösti sounds so much more, you know, rococo. Try them canapé-sized at your next canasta tournament.

Serves 4
counts towards your 5-a-day

2 waxy potatoes (Desiree are
    good)
2 apples (Cox's or Granny
    Smiths work really well)
juice of 1 lemon
a small handful of grated
    cheese (Cheddar, Cheshire
    or Wensleydale)
plain flour
olive oil

Peel the potatoes and put them into a large pan of boiling water. Bring back to the boil and cook for about 8 minutes – you just want to take the edge off their rawness. Drain them in a colander and set aside to steam and cool off.

Meanwhile, grate the apples into a bowl and toss them in the lemon juice.

Once the potatoes have cooled, grate them into the bowl. Then use your hands to squeeze any excess liquid out of the mixture.

Stir in most of the cheese, season with salt and pepper, and shape the mixture into flat cakes. Don't worry about being too neat – the rough bits will go all crispy when you cook them. Dust the cakes with flour, sprinkle with the remaining cheese and pop them into the fridge until you're ready to cook them.

Preheat your oven to 200°C/400°F/gas mark 6.

Drizzle a baking tray with olive oil or line with greaseproof paper, pop the rösti on to it and drizzle them with oil too. Bake in the oven for 10 minutes, then flip them over and cook for another 10 minutes, until golden and crispy on both sides.

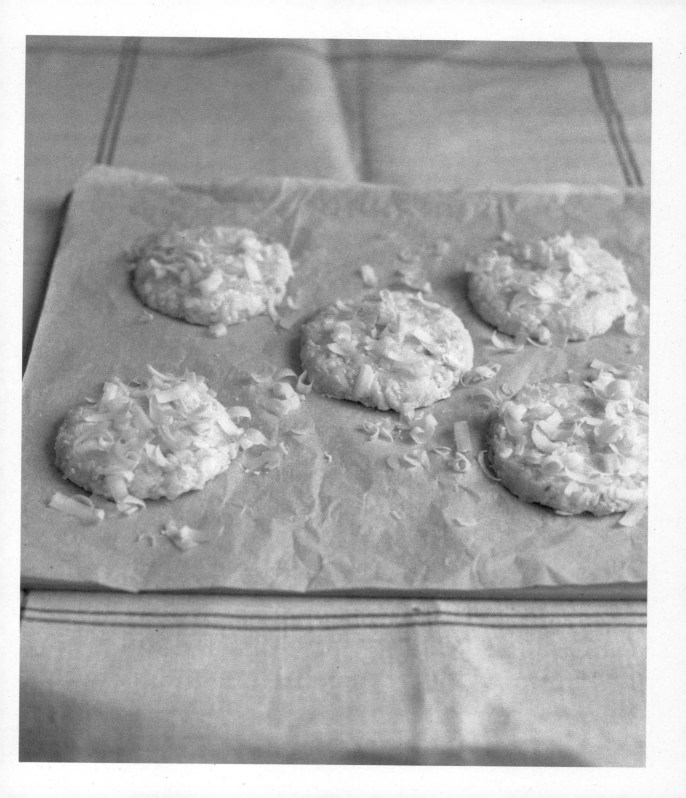

# Eat Your
# GREENS
# AND REDS
## YELLOWS, ORANGES AND
## PURPLES TOO

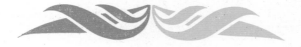

Variety is the spice of life.

And when it comes to fruit
and veg, the more you mix it
up colourwise, the better.

If you only eat carrots, you'll get
bored, stop being invited out to
dinner and maybe turn orange.

So, by eating a spectrum
of different coloured fruit and
veg, you'll reap the benefits of
all the nutrients that Mother
Nature thoughtfully distributed
between them and go to
dinner parties more often.

# Lebanese lentil salad

Nutty Puy lentils, toasted pumpkin seeds, a bashing of spices and sweet, sweet pomegranate – it's like an exotic disco in your mouth (if discos came dusted with sumac and with flatbreads on the side). Oh look. There's Bianca Jagger on a white horse.

Serves 4
2 portions of your 5-a-day

1 pomegranate
a small bunch of parsley, stalks removed, leaves roughly chopped
a small bunch of mint, stalks removed, leaves roughly chopped
1 x 400g tin of Puy lentils, drained
a big handful of cherry tomatoes, quartered
2 roasted red peppers from a jar, roughly chopped
a handful of toasted pumpkin seeds
4 flatbreads
extra virgin olive oil
a pinch of sumac
1 teaspoon coriander seeds, bashed up
1 teaspoon cumin seeds, bashed up
juice of ½ a lime
juice of ½ an orange
1 teaspoon honey

Heat your grill to medium.

Cut the pomegranate in half and hold one half over a small bowl. Tap the outside with a wooden spoon and allow the seeds (known as jewels) to tumble into the bowl. Then do the same with the other half.

In a big bowl, mix together the chopped herbs, lentils, tomatoes, red peppers, pumpkin seeds and half the pomegranate seeds.

Drizzle the flatbreads with a little olive oil, sprinkle with sumac, and toast under the grill for a couple of minutes.

Put the bashed-up coriander and cumin seeds into a frying pan over a medium heat and toast for a minute or so. Add a good drizzle of olive oil, the lime juice, orange juice and honey and cook for a couple of minutes, until reduced down.

Pour the warm dressing over the lentils, give them a good stir, top with the rest of the pomegranate seeds and serve immediately with the toasted flatbreads.

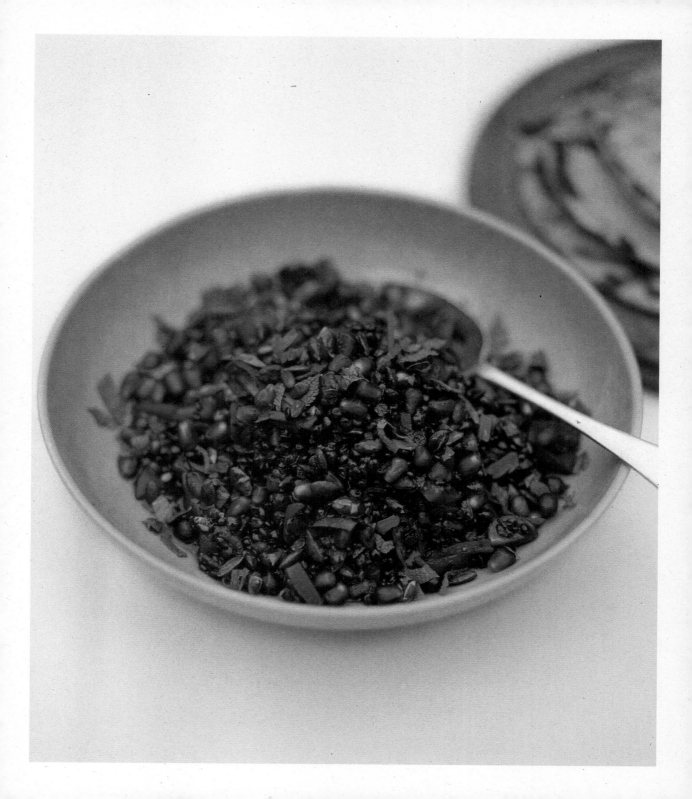

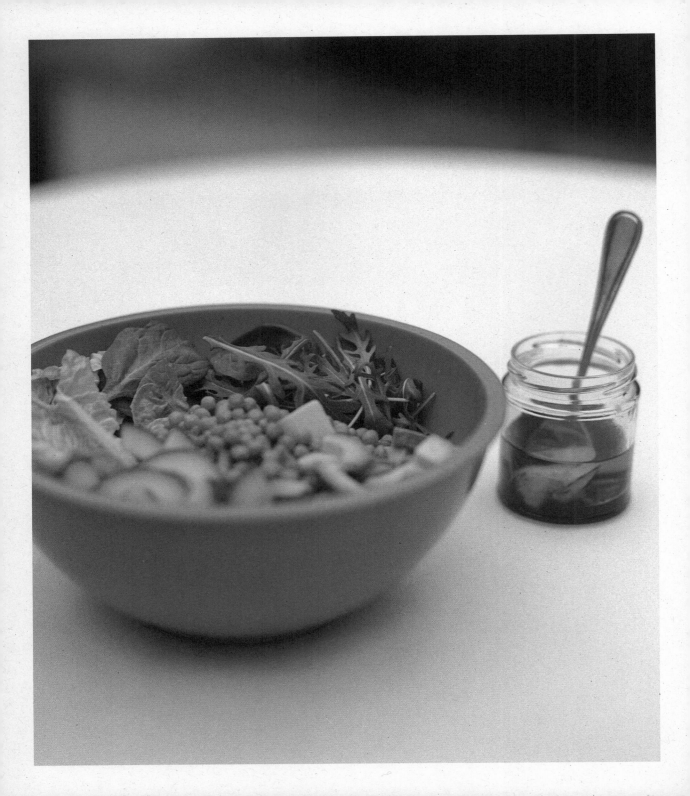

# Green salad

**Lettuce plus friends transforms a sad excuse for a salad into a party on a plate. And you're invited.**

Serves 4
3 portions of your 5-a-day

For the salad

2 little gem lettuces
2 big handfuls of spinach
2 big handfuls of rocket or
  watercress
½ a cucumber
2 handfuls of fresh peas or
  cooked frozen peas
1 avocado

For the dressing

3 tablespoons olive oil
1 tablespoon balsamic
  vinegar
1 teaspoon Dijon mustard

Break off the little gem leaves and wash them with the spinach and rocket in a sink of cold water. Remove the excess water by either popping your leaves into a salad spinner or drying them carefully in a clean tea-towel. Once dried, put them into a big salad bowl.

Slice the cucumber in half down the middle and use a teaspoon to scoop out the seeds. Then slice into half moons and add to the bowl along with the peas. Peel the avocado and remove the stone, then chop the flesh into small chunks. Add to the bowl, toss together and set to one side.

Put all the dressing ingredients into a jam jar, season well and give it a good shake. Any leftover dressing will keep in the fridge for at least a week.

To serve, drizzle some dressing over the salad and toss again.

# THINGS TO DO IN 30 Minutes

While you're waiting for the cake to bake

Leave your street the normal way ➡ Turn right keep going then take 2nd left ⬅ Walk for (5) minutes exactly ➡ Turn right again and leave a pound coin (£1) on the pavement for the next lucky person to find

Watch an episode of something

RUN!

GIVE THE DOG A BATH
(5 minutes to bathe him, 20 minutes to catch him)

(5 minutes to let him dry off)

GET YOUR PING-PONG ON

BBRRIING! BBRRIING!

HELLO?

LEARN TO PLAY CHESS

BURY A

TIME CAPSULE

IN THE GARDEN

Call someone you haven't spoken to for ages. Or someone you usually speak to when you're doing something else and give them your full and undivided attention.

PLANT A VEGETABLE PATCH

HELP OUT AN OLDER PERSON

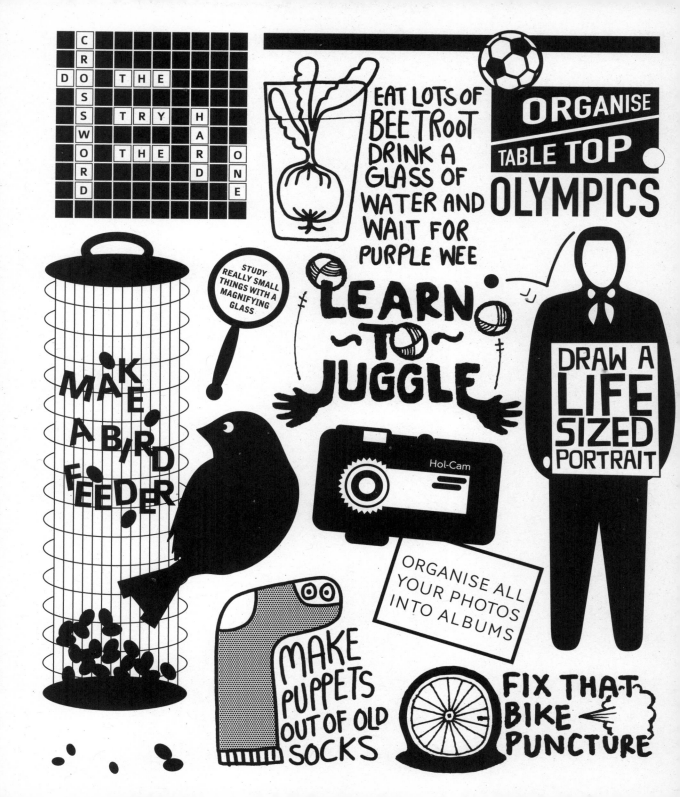

# Rainbow coleslaw

(To the tune of 'I Can Sing a Rainbow'.)

*Red and orange and pink and green,*
*Lemony yoghurty jus.*
*Here's a cabbage rainbow,*
*Cabbage rainbow,*
*With some pine nuts too.*

Serves 4
1½ portions of your 5-a-day

½ a small red cabbage
1 head of spring greens,
   or pointed or sweetheart
   cabbage
a handful of radishes
4 spring onions
3 carrots
2 apples
zest and juice of 1 lemon
4 tablespoons plain yoghurt
   or crème fraîche
extra virgin olive oil

Finely shred the cabbages and put into a big bowl. Finely slice the radishes and spring onions and add to the bowl.

Peel the carrots and grate into the bowl, then grate in the apples, leaving the skins on. Mix everything together well.

Stir in the lemon zest and juice, then add the yoghurt or crème fraîche and a good glug of olive oil. Give it all another mix and season.

This is great on its own, or on top of a burger, a baked potato or with a slice of your favourite cheese and a hunk of granary bread for a super-quick lunch.

Add a sprinkling of toasted seeds, pine nuts or raisins for a crunchy treat.

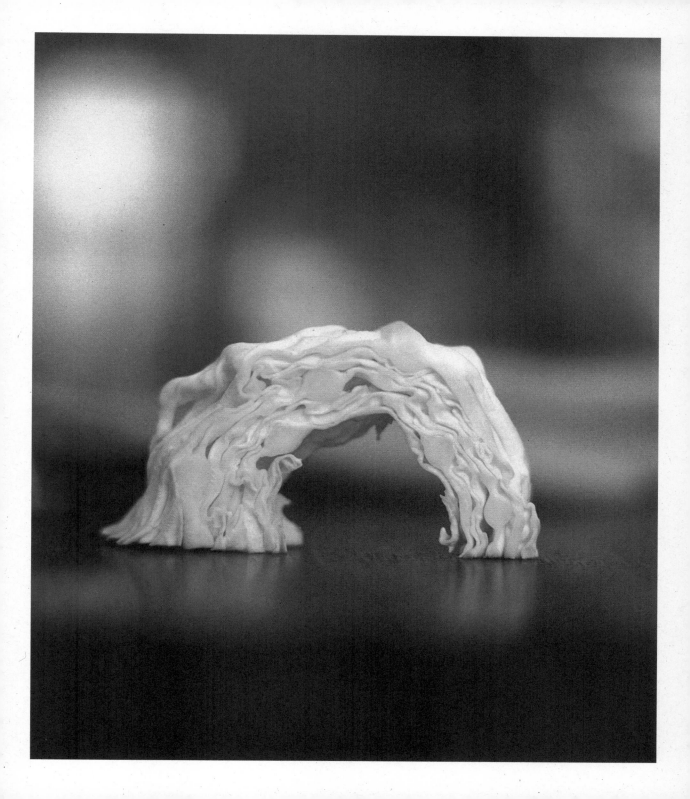

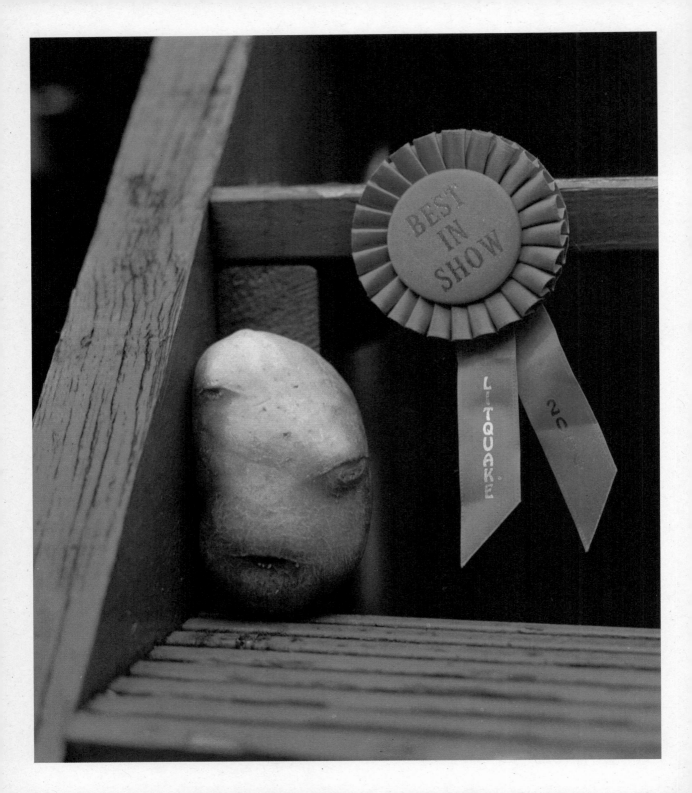

# Best potato salad

Highly commended in the St Catherine's Church Allotment Show, Newcastle upon Tyne, 1994, and best in show at Litquake 2004, this is a winner of a recipe. If you can't get your hands on Jersey Royals or new potatoes, you can use waxy spuds like Desirée instead. Just make sure you boil them for a little longer.

**Serves 4**

800g Jersey Royals or new
    potatoes, quartered
a few sprigs of basil, roughly
    chopped
a few sprigs of mint, roughly
    chopped
a few sprigs of parsley,
    roughly chopped
1 tablespoon capers, roughly
    chopped
2 tablespoons mayonnaise
2 tablespoons plain yoghurt
    or crème fraîche
juice of 1 lemon
1 teaspoon mustard
1 teaspoon runny honey

Put the potatoes into a pan, cover with cold water and bring to the boil. Turn down the heat and allow to simmer for 10 to 12 minutes, until tender. Turn off the heat, drain, cover and leave to one side.

Next, mix the chopped herbs and capers in a bowl with the mayo, yoghurt or crème fraîche, lemon juice, mustard and honey. Season and check the balance of flavours, adding a bit more lemon, mustard or honey as needed.

Put the potatoes in a serving dish and pour the dressing over them while they are still warm, so they soak up the flavours, then toss everything together and serve straight away.

# Robot food

In this age of iStuff, Large Hadron Colliders and push-up bras, we have never been closer to The World of Tomorrow. Whatever will be next? Hoverboots? Telekinetic dogs? Well no, actually, it's robots. Before long, diligent and charmingly British robots will be living with us, doing our chores whilst we laze about in silver jumpsuits waiting for the moon bus. This recipe is for when that happens. Remember, keep your robot fed. Otherwise he'll try and find his own food. And this could result in either a messy kitchen or you being eaten.

Serves 1.0
100% RDA of heavy metals

95kg chipped aluminium
1 family sized bag of diodes, LEDs are best if you can get them
1 metre of normal housing wiring, the more colours the better
a generous handful of those small, round, silver batteries that go in watches
1 lightbulb
2.5 litres engine oil
a pinch or two of cracked black pepper and sea salt
1 Etch A Sketch®'s worth of iron filings

Preheat your oven to 375,000°C/675,000°F/gas mark 2000. Take your aluminium out of the fridge. You can use the normal stuff or, if you're feeling fancy, go for brushed.

Next, combine your diodes, wires and batteries in a large bowl. Crack in your lightbulb and stir whilst slowly adding the oil.

When your mixture is a consistent metallic dough, remove from the bowl and roll out on a reinforced steel worktop. Take your aluminium chips and lay them out evenly on the top of your rolled dough.

Put on a welder's mask and flame-retardant gloves and open the oven door. Carefully put your dressed slab on to the top shelf of the oven (remember your dish will weigh more than a large boy, so lift with your knees). Let it all bake for about 2 hours, or until the aluminium has formed a white-hot molten crust.

When it's ready, remove from the oven and place in your cryogenic storage freezer. If you don't have one, put it on the windowsill for a month and a half. Once cooled, cut into thin strips of exactly 16.3mm x 33.7mm. For this you'll need an industrial girder saw and a ruler.

Finally, arrange your strips in a newspaper cone, season with salt, pepper and iron filings to taste and serve.

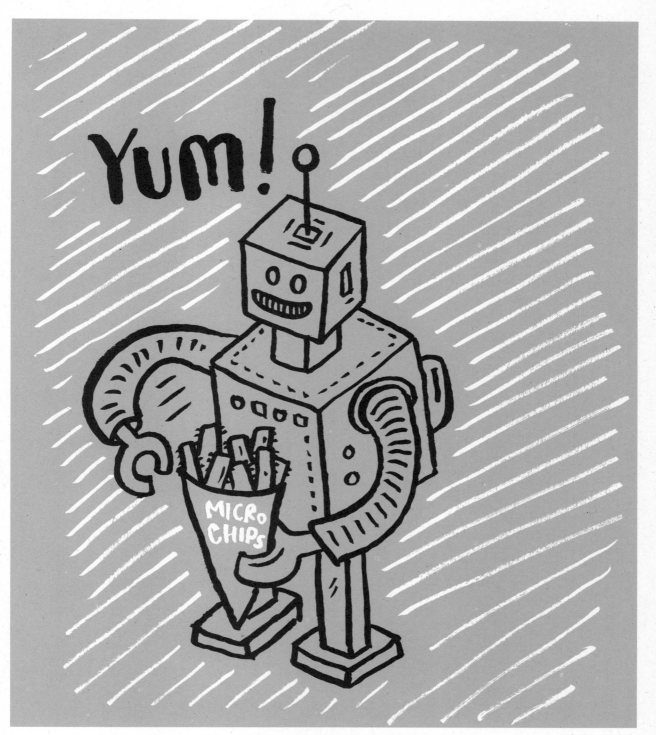

'01110100 01100001 01110011 01110100 01111001.'

# Chop chop salad

We recommend using a sharp knife for this recipe. You can, of course, try using the side of your hand. Granted, it might get tricky around the tomato stage. But it's your salad. And you'll chop it how you like.

Serves 4
1½ portions of your 5-a-day

**For the salad**
½ a cucumber
1 carrot, peeled
4 radishes
1 tomato
1 spring onion
1 little gem lettuce
a small bunch of mint
a very small handful of poppy
   seeds
a small handful of pumpkin
   seeds, toasted

**For the dressing**
1 teaspoon mustard
½ teaspoon runny honey
a splash of red wine vinegar
a bigger splash of extra virgin
   olive oil

First find a massive chopping board.

Put the cucumber, carrot and radishes on the board and roughly chop them. Move them to one side.

Put the tomato, spring onion, little gem and mint leaves on the board and chop those.

Then get a big knife and chop everything together, using a rocking motion, until it is all mixed and very well chopped. Pop it into a salad serving bowl.

Put all the dressing ingredients into a jam jar and shake well.

Pour the dressing over the salad, season and sprinkle with the seeds. Eat straight away. Otherwise it'll go all soggy. Which is not salad cricket.

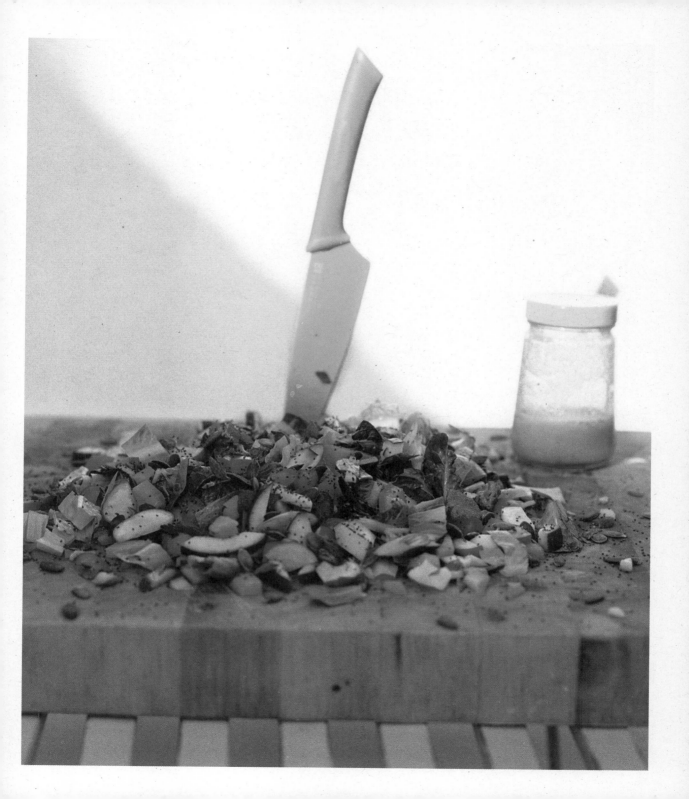

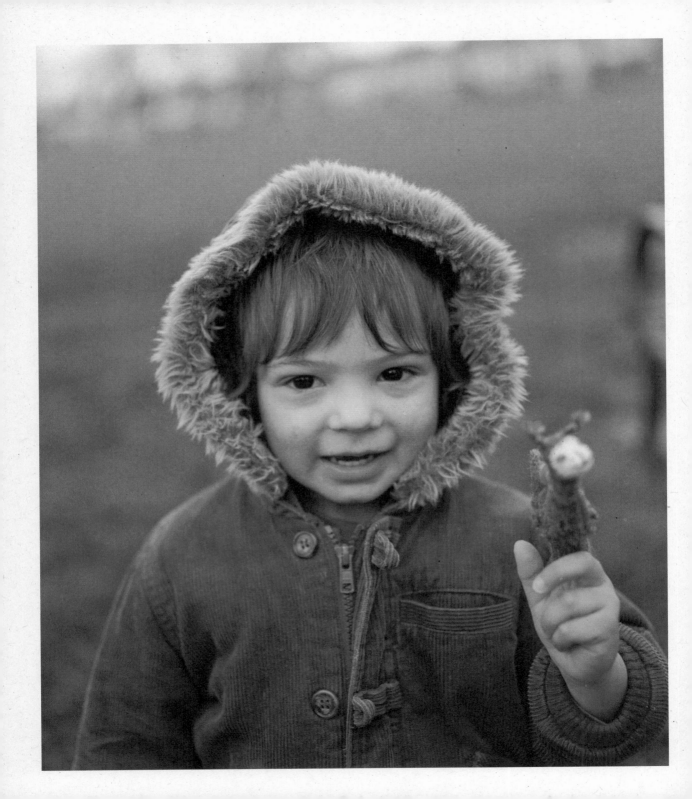

# Green quinoa salad

Pronounced *keen-wah*, this nutty little grain often gets pooh-poohed as the fodder of yuppie dinner parties and weirdy-beardy health food shops. It is, in fact, an extremely versatile and delicious, lighter alternative to couscous. And the Aztecs used to eat it for breakfast, lunch and dinner. And they knew a thing or two, them Aztecs.

Serves 4

1 portion of your 5-a-day

2 mugs of quinoa (400g)
4 mugs of water
1 chicken or vegetable stock
  cube, crumbled
1 large head of broccoli, cut
  into bite-sized florets
a bunch of asparagus spears,
  woody ends removed, cut
  into bite-sized pieces
a small bunch of basil
a small bunch of mint
a handful of toasted almonds
extra virgin olive oil
3 big handfuls of spinach
200g feta cheese, crumbled
a handful of toasted seeds
1 lemon, cut into wedges

Put the quinoa into a pan and cover with the water. Crumble in the stock cube and bring to the boil, then reduce the heat and leave to simmer for about 10 minutes, until most of the water has been absorbed. Just before all the water is absorbed, remove from the heat, add half of the broccoli and all the asparagus, cover with a lid and allow to steam for 3 to 4 minutes.

While the quinoa is cooking, put the rest of the broccoli florets into a food processor with all the basil, mint, toasted almonds and a good drizzle of olive oil and whizz until it looks like a kind of pesto.

Then fluff up the quinoa with a fork and stir in the pesto dressing.

Serve with fresh spinach, topped with feta and toasted seeds and the lemon wedges, for squeezing.

# Rainbow chips

**Chips made healthy. And colourful. Naturally. Woo hoo.**

1 carrot
1 parsnip
1 potato
2 sweet potatoes
1 large beetroot
1 courgette
olive oil

Preheat your oven to 200°C/400°F/gas mark 6.

Peel the carrot and parsnip, and scrub the potato, sweet potatoes and beetroot. Cut all the vegetables, including the courgette, into long chip-shaped pieces.

Bring a large pan of water to the boil. Add the carrot, parsnip, potato and sweet potatoes, bring back to the boil, and cook for about 5 minutes. Drain and leave to drip dry in a colander.

Lay all the vegetables on a baking tray (use 2 if necessary). Drizzle with olive oil, season well with salt and pepper, and toss till the veg are well coated.

Bake in the oven for 30 minutes, until the veg are golden brown and crispy round the edges. Serve with a big dollop of homemade traffic-light ketchup (page 310).

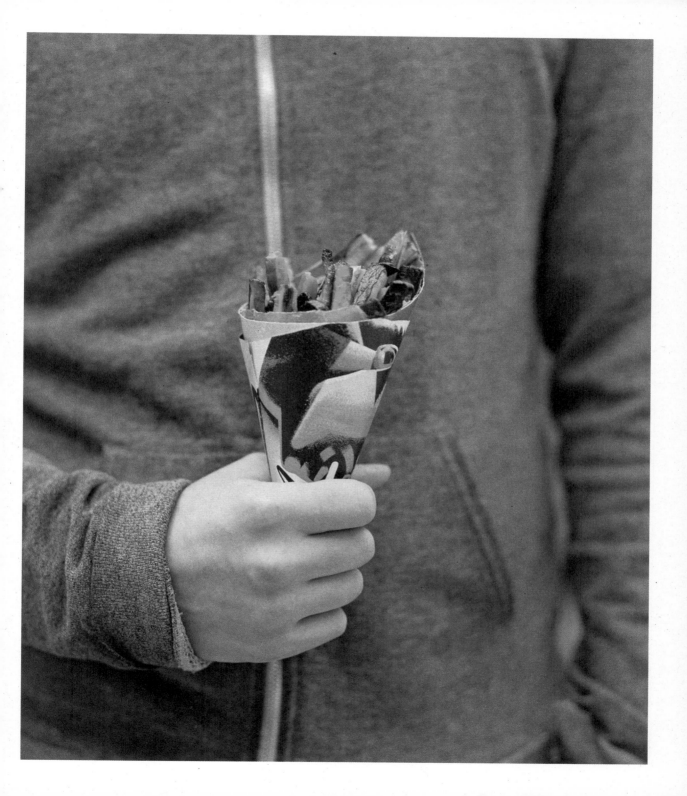

# Some classic sides

Here's a few more side dishes to make your plate even more jazzy and vegetably. All these recipes serve 4 and are 1 portion of your 5-a-day.

### Simple spinach

Melt a knob of butter in a large pan and chuck in 500g of fresh spinach. Add a tablespoon of water and cook over a medium heat for a few minutes, until the spinach starts to wilt. Stir in some freshly grated nutmeg and season well. Take off the heat, add a splash of single cream, and serve.

### Roasted broccoli

Preheat your oven to 180°C/350°F/gas mark 4.

Chop a big head of broccoli into bite-sized florets, toss in a drizzle of olive oil and roast for 20 minutes.

Then finely chop ½ a red chilli and 2 cloves of garlic. Finely grate a small knob of ginger and mix the lot into the broccoli. Roast for another 20 minutes until golden and crispy. Just before serving, drizzle with a little honey and soy sauce.

### Creamed corn

Cut the kernels off 4 cobs of corn, add them to a pan with a little knob of butter and cook slowly for 10 minutes. Mash up with a potato masher, add a little splash of single cream and season. Bring to a simmer and serve.

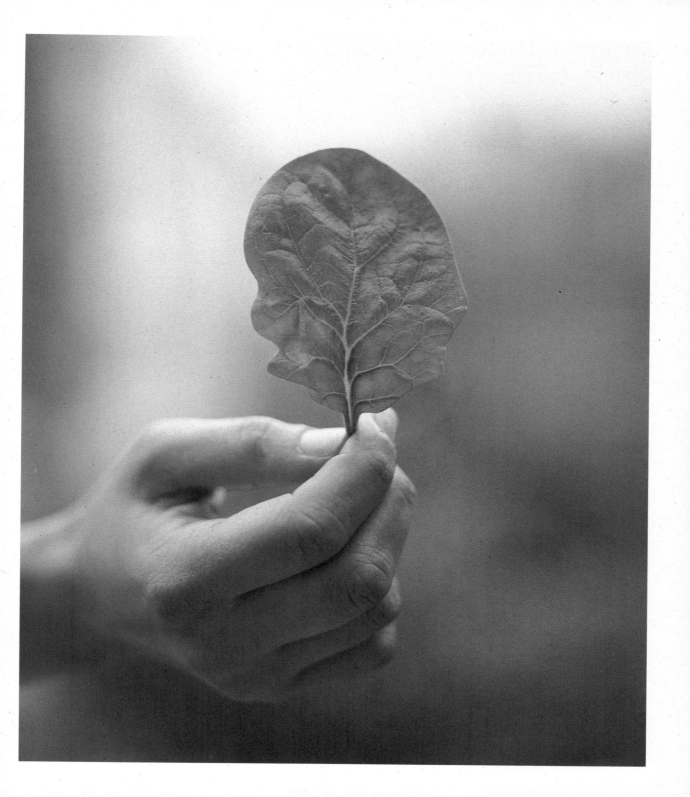

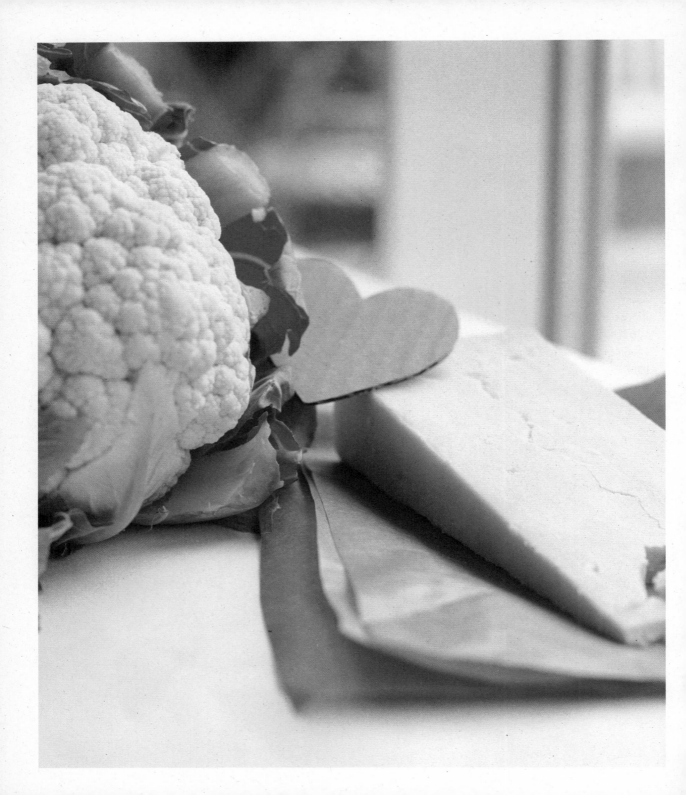

# Cauliflower cheese

You've had this before, haven't you? At school probably. After double chemistry, when you sat next to that kid with the elastic band in his teeth. Well this one is better than the one you had at school.

Serves 4
1 portion of your 5-a-day

1 litre milk
1 bay leaf
1 small onion, peeled and cut into wedges
2 cloves
1 large cauliflower
50g butter
3 tablespoons plain flour
100g mature Cheddar cheese, grated

Preheat your oven to 180°C/350°F/gas mark 4.

Put the milk into a pan with the bay leaf, onion and cloves and bring to the boil, making sure it doesn't boil over. Once bubbling, turn off the heat, remove the onion, bay leaf and cloves and allow the milk to sit for a few minutes.

Break the cauliflower into bite-sized florets and cut the stalk into thin slices. Put it all in a pan, cover with boiling water, bring to the boil and simmer for 3 minutes. Drain, then set aside in a colander and allow to dry off.

Add the butter to the pan and let it melt over a low heat, then stir in the flour and cook for a couple of minutes, until it starts to brown. Add the hot milk gradually, beating as you go, until you have added all the milk. Don't worry if there are a few little lumps. You can always bash them out or put the sauce through a sieve.

Once you're happy with the sauce, stir in most of the cheese. Put the cauliflower into a baking dish, pour over the cheese sauce, top with a little more grated cheese and bake in the hot oven for 20 to 25 minutes, until golden.

# Honey and Parmesan parsnips

**The toast of all good roasts. Caramelise with gay abandon.**

Serves 4
1 portion of your 5-a-day

8 parsnips, peeled and cut
    into long thin quarters
olive oil
clear honey, for drizzling
a few sprigs of thyme, stalks
    removed
100g freshly grated Parmesan
    cheese

Preheat the oven to 200°C/400°F/gas mark 6.

Place the parsnips in a pan of boiling water, bring back to the boil and cook for 5 minutes. Drain in a colander for a couple of minutes to allow any excess water to drip out.

Put the parsnips on to a baking tray, drizzle with olive oil and honey, and sprinkle with the thyme leaves. Give everything a good shuffle around and roast in the oven for 25 minutes.

After 25 minutes, take the parsnips out of the oven and scatter over the Parmesan. Stir the parsnips around so that they are well coated. Then pop them back into the oven for another 10 minutes or so, until golden and caramelised.

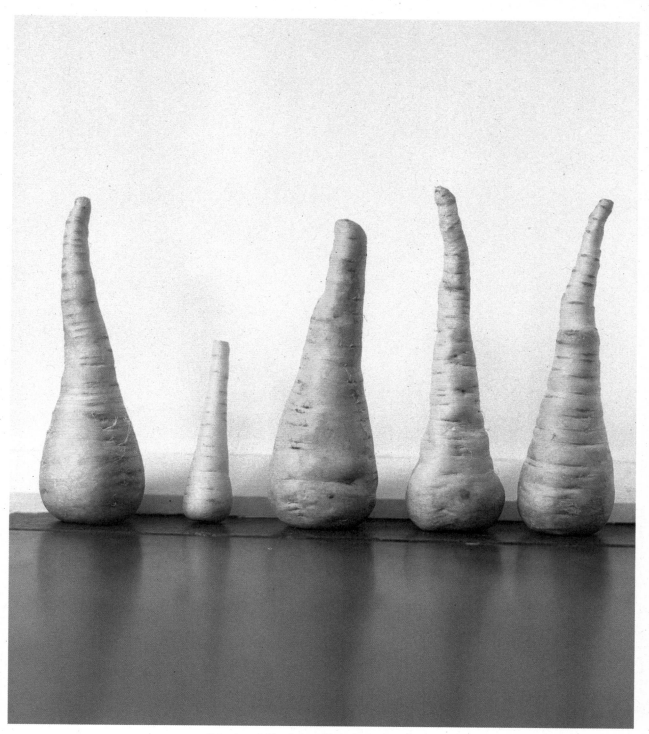

'Number 4. That's him. He stole my handbag.'

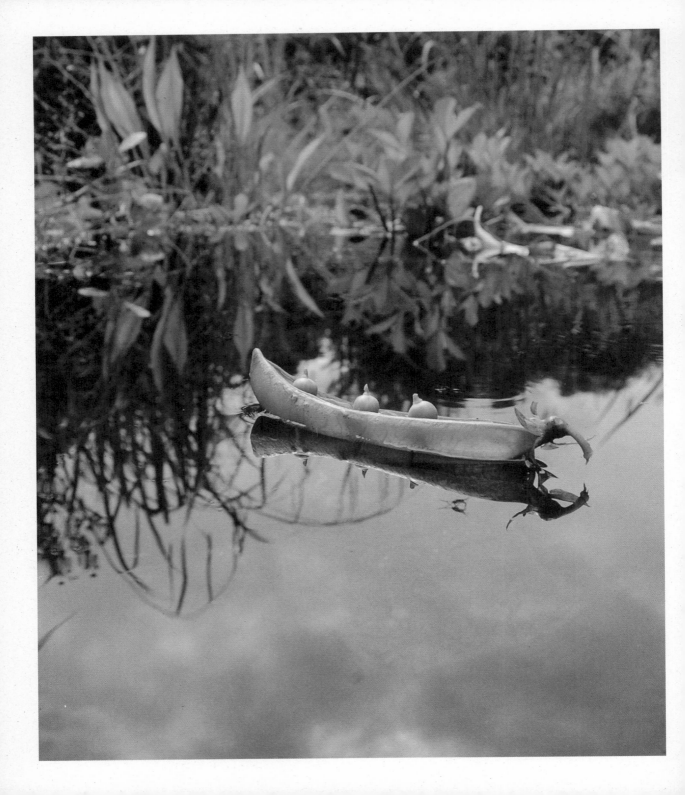

# QUICK THINGS TO DO WITH

---

# VEG

Boiled is boring. And takes all the goodness out of your veg (with the exception of carrots, which are more nutritious when cooked. But we digress...).

Here are a load more quick and easy ideas to jazz up your veg, bump up your daily portion, and rejuvenate any overcooked cauliflower to leftover glory:

**Dip it.** Cut up your favourite veg into sticks and serve with quick tomato salsa (page 103), plain yoghurt with torn basil or smoked paprika, a blob of peanut butter or a homemade dip (page 106).

**Grated carrot or shredded spinach** in sandwiches works really well.

**Leftover veg?** Mash it up, shape into little patties with a drizzle of olive oil and then lightly fry or grill for a tasty snack.

**Try eating vegetables like fruit.** A whole pepper or tomato for instance. If you've got a juicer, try adding the odd carrot or beetroot to your favourite juice for an added veggie hit.

And turn the page for even more great ways to cook your veg. All the recipes that follow will serve 4 as a side dish.

# Aubergines

Here are a load of things to do with eggplants (please note, none of the following recipes contains eggs).

### Mozzarella and pesto

Cut an aubergine in half lengthways and put into a roasting tray. Drizzle with olive oil, season with salt and pepper and roast in the oven at 200°C/400°F/gas mark 6 for about 30 minutes. Take out of the oven and top each half with a tablespoon of pesto and a few blobs of mozzarella. Pop back into the oven for 5 minutes, until the cheese melts and starts to bubble. Serves 2 as a main meal with a green salad or 4 as a side dish.

### Souk style

Cut an aubergine into cubes, season with salt and pepper and roast in the oven at 200°C/400°F/gas mark 6 for about 20 minutes, until golden. Pop the aubergine into a bowl and toss with freshly chopped mint, a little bit of crumbled feta cheese and a handful of pomegranate seeds to make a warm and tasty salad. Serve piled on top of salad leaves.

### Miso aubergine

Cut an aubergine in half lengthways and put into a roasting tray. Roast in the oven at 200°C/400°F/gas mark 6 for about 30 minutes. Make a quick dressing using a tablespoon each of miso paste, soy sauce and runny honey. Pour over the roasted aubergine and return it to the oven for a few minutes. Great with rice and steamed greens.

### Red aubergine

Chop an aubergine into big chunks and fry in a lightly oiled pan until golden. Add a tin of tomatoes, a splash of red wine vinegar and some torn-up basil and simmer for 10 minutes. Serve stirred into pasta, with a little grating of Parmesan, or on its own as a side dish.

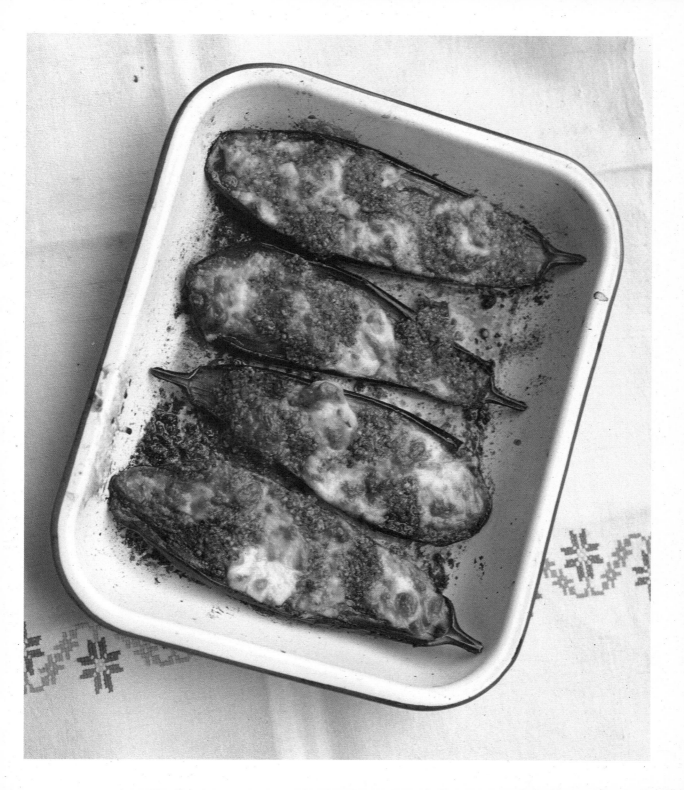

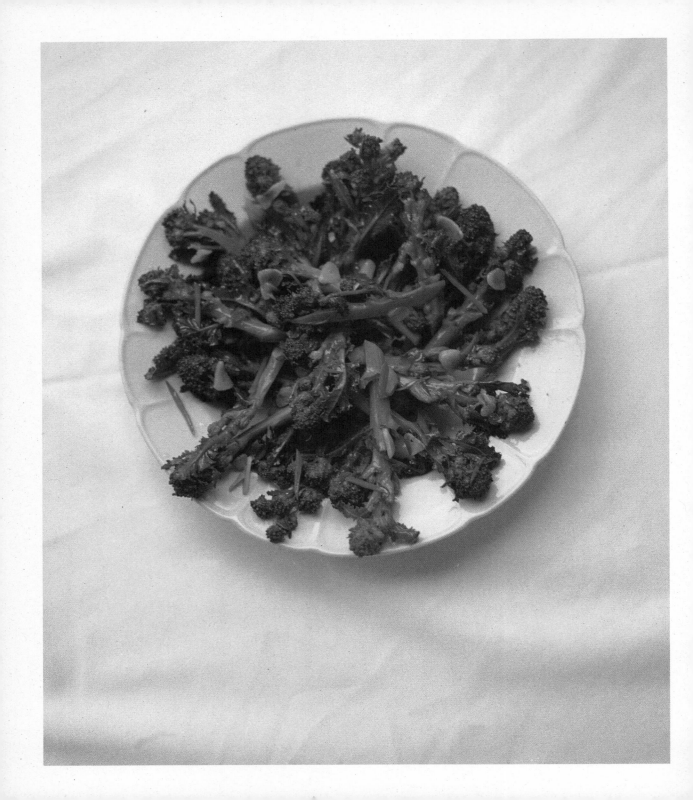

# Broccoli

A brassica proverb:

*If you steam, your broccoli will always be tender and green.*
*If you boil the living daylights out of it, no one will eat it.*

This is the way of the broccoli.

## Honey and soy

Steam 1 head of broccoli florets for a couple of minutes so they're still bright green with a bit of bite. Then fry 2 peeled and finely chopped cloves of garlic and a thumb-sized piece of peeled and grated ginger in a little oil. Add the steamed broccoli, stir-fry for a couple of minutes, then add a drizzle of honey and a splash of soy sauce.

## Italian style

Finely chop a couple of cloves of peeled garlic and ½ a red chilli and fry for a couple of minutes in a drizzle of olive oil. Chop up 1 head of broccoli and add to the pan with a splash of water. You can add a couple of anchovies if you like – you won't taste them, think of them as a seasoning. Cook for about 10 minutes, until the broccoli starts to break down. Great stirred through pasta.

## Broccoli cheese

Just replace the cauliflower with broccoli (page 229).

## Posh broc

Toast a handful of flaked almonds in a pan and add a handful of raisins and a little knob of butter. Cook for a couple of minutes, then pour over steamed broccoli, give it a good stir and serve.

# Beetroots

Turn your wee pink, your hair orange and your plate colourful. Beet that for a root veg with excellent added side effects.

### Boiled beets

Boil beetroots in salted water for 30 to 40 minutes, depending on their size, or until a knife goes through them easily. Allow to cool, then peel them (you may want to use gloves as they stain your hands) and keep them in the fridge to use in salads, sandwiches or red hummus (page 106).

### Roasted beets

Boil 10 beetroots in salted water for 20 to 30 minutes, depending on how big they are. Allow to cool, then peel off the skins, cut in half, and put into a roasting tray with some olive oil, salt, pepper, a splash of wine vinegar and a few sprigs of thyme. Roast at 180°C/350°F/gas mark 4 for 20 minutes.

### Spiced beets

Cut up 4 cooked and peeled beetroots. Heat a pinch of cumin and coriander seed in a pan, then bash in a pestle and mortar and add to the beets with a little orange juice, some olive oil and a pinch of salt and pepper.

### Hot pink beets

Grate raw peeled beetroots into a bowl and dress with lemon juice, a spoonful of plain yoghurt and a pinch of salt and pepper for a super-quick kind of hot pink coleslaw.

# Cabbage

Red, white, pointy, Savoy, Chinese – so many cabbages, so little time. Better get shredding.

### Sweet red

Finely shred ½ a red cabbage. Heat a little olive oil in a pan, add the cabbage, a couple of chopped apples and a good splash of balsamic vinegar, and cook on a medium heat for 20 minutes, until the cabbage is soft and sweet.

### Chinese white cabbage

Shred ½ a white cabbage and cook it in boiling salted water for a few minutes, until tender. Drain and put in a serving dish. Top with oyster sauce, chopped chilli and chopped coriander and toss together.

### Savoy cabbage

Shred ½ a Savoy cabbage and cook it in boiling salted water for a couple of minutes, until just tender. Drain. Heat a little butter in a pan and add a pinch of fennel seeds and if you like some lardons; once these are golden, add the cabbage and toss to coat.

### Black cabbage

Use cavolo nero when you can get it, and when you can't, kale will do fine. Steam or blanch 4 handfuls of greens, then drain and add a little olive oil to the pan along with 2 peeled and crushed garlic cloves. Cook for a couple of minutes, then throw in the greens and a sprinkling of lemon zest. Grate Parmesan over before serving.

# Carrots

Renowned in the UK for helping people to see in the dark, famed in France for cheering up the grumpy, the carrot is the finest pointy vegetable in the universe. With parsnips a very close second.

### Seedy carrot salad

Peel and grate 4 carrots into a bowl. Toast a handful of sunflower and pumpkin seeds with a pinch of cumin seeds and add to the bowl. Stir in 2 tablespoons of plain yoghurt and a squeeze of lemon juice, season well and mix the whole lot together.

### Baked orangey carrots

Peel 6 carrots and finely slice lengthways. Pop them into an ovenproof dish with a splash of orange juice, a little knob of butter and some salt and pepper. Cover with foil and bake in the oven at 200°C/400°F/ gas mark 6 for 25 minutes. Great with roast dinner.

### Little carrot fritters

Grate 4 carrots into a bowl and add 1 tablespoon of plain flour, 1 peeled and crushed garlic clove and a handful of roughly chopped coriander. Mix together and make into little cakes. Either lightly fry in a drizzle of olive oil or pop under the grill on a piece of foil for a couple of minutes (remembering to flip) on each side until golden.

### Spicy carrots

Scrub 10 carrots and chop in half lengthways. Put them into a pan of boiling lightly salted water for a couple of minutes, then drain and pop them into a roasting tin along with a drizzle of olive oil, 2 teaspoons of crushed coriander seeds and some seasoning. Roast for 30 minutes at 180°C/350°F/gas mark 4 and serve with a blob of plain yoghurt.

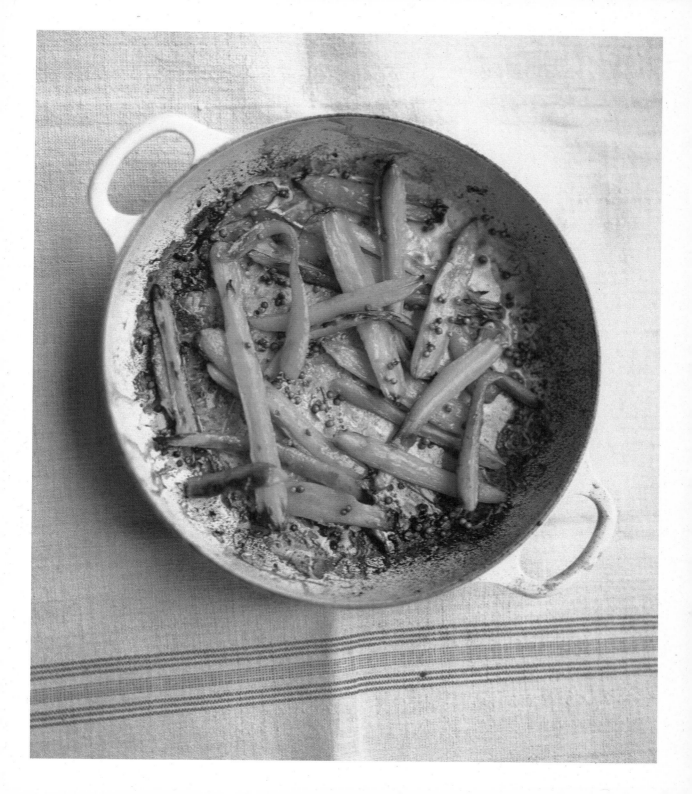

# Cauliflower

Looks like it came from outer space, tastes out of this world (especially when paired with cheese, spices or a little yoghurty dressing).

### Spicy roast cauliflower

Cut 1 medium head of cauliflower into florets and steam or boil until just tender. Drain and pop into a baking dish along with a pinch of garam masala, a drizzle of olive oil and some salt and pepper. Bake at 200°C/400°F/gas mark 6 for 25 minutes, until just golden. Once roasted, add a squeeze of lemon, a spoonful of plain yoghurt and a sprinkling of roughly chopped fresh coriander. Serve with plain rice and mango chutney for a quick dinner.

### Cauliflower salad

Chop ½ a head of cauliflower into little florets and pop into a bowl with the juice of ½ a lemon, a spoonful of plain yoghurt and some chopped dill or parsley. Mix together and serve with a sprinkling of toasted seeds.

### Spanish cauliflower

Cut 1 medium head of cauliflower into florets and steam or boil until just tender. Drain and add to a pan with a drizzle of olive oil and a pinch of smoked paprika. Lightly fry until golden, then stir in some capers and a sprinkling of chopped parsley.

Looking for a cheesy version? You just went past it. It's on page 229.

# Courgettes

The oblong-ish relative of the oddly-shaped-anyway squash family, courgettes taste as good grated, fried or soused in tomato as they do lightly griddled with a squeeze of lemon and a hint of chilli.

## Ribbon salad

Use the thin slicing attachment on a food processor to peel 4 courgettes into long ribbons. Or use a bog-standard potato peeler. Pop the courgette ribbons into a bowl with the juice of ½ a lemon, a handful of roughly chopped mint or basil and a drizzle of olive oil. Mix together and season well.

For a simple supper, serve with a little crumbled goat's cheese and a hunk of bread. Or have as a side dish.

## Red courgettes

Chop 4 courgettes into small chunks and fry in a lightly oiled pan for 10 minutes until soft. Add a 400g tin of chopped tomatoes or 3 chopped fresh ones and continue to cook for another 5 minutes or so. Finally, add some torn-up basil, season well and serve. This works really well with a little crumbled feta.

## Chilli lemon courgettes

Heat up a griddle pan. Slice 4 courgettes into long strips or coins, and grill on the dry griddle until nicely charred on both sides. Add to a bowl with a squeeze of lemon juice, a drizzle of olive oil, a small handful of fresh mint and some finely chopped red chilli, and give it a good mix before seasoning.

## Dill courgettes

Chop 4 courgettes into coins and fry in a lightly oiled pan with a couple of peeled and crushed garlic cloves. Cook until golden, and serve with a small handful of chopped dill.

# Green beans

**Lean, green, beany machines – climb aboard and steam away.**

### Red beans

Steam a pack of green beans until just tender. Stir in 2 tablespoons of tomato purée and sprinkle with a little grated Parmesan. Bingo.

### Cheesy beans

Steam a pack of green beans until just tender and grate or crumble in a little of your favourite melty cheese (Taleggio, brie or Cheddar). The heat of the beans will melt the cheese, but you can always pop it into the oven for 5 minutes if you want it really melty. Leave it another 2 minutes for a crunchy topping.

### French beans

Steam your beans until just tender and toss with a little knob of butter, a squeeze of lemon juice and some very finely chopped shallots.

### Sweet beans

Steam your beans until just tender. Mix together 1 teaspoon of grainy mustard, 1 teaspoon of honey, a little splash of chilli sauce and 1 tablespoon of olive oil. Toss the warm beans in the dressing and serve steaming.

# Peas

Spherically perfect. The emerald pearls of the veg world. And very annoying to eat if your kitchen happens to be on a slant.

## Mushy peas

Cook 4 handfuls of frozen peas in boiling salted water, then drain and return them to the pan. Add a small handful of chopped mint, the juice of ½ a lemon, a little knob of butter and some salt and pepper. Mash with a fork and eat with fish, on toast or stirred through pasta.

## French peas

Finely chop 1 leek and cook in a little butter until soft. Add 4 handfuls of frozen peas and about 100ml veg or chicken stock, and simmer until the peas are cooked. Add 2 shredded little gem lettuces and stir-fry until wilted. Season well and serve.

## Posh peas

Cook 4 handfuls of frozen peas in boiling salted water, then drain and return to the pan. Leave to cool. Mix a small handful of chopped basil, some crumbled feta and some rocket or watercress in a bowl. Add the peas, a squeeze of lemon juice and a drizzle of olive oil. Serve with quinoa, couscous or a hunk of wholemeal bread for a quick, fresh supper.

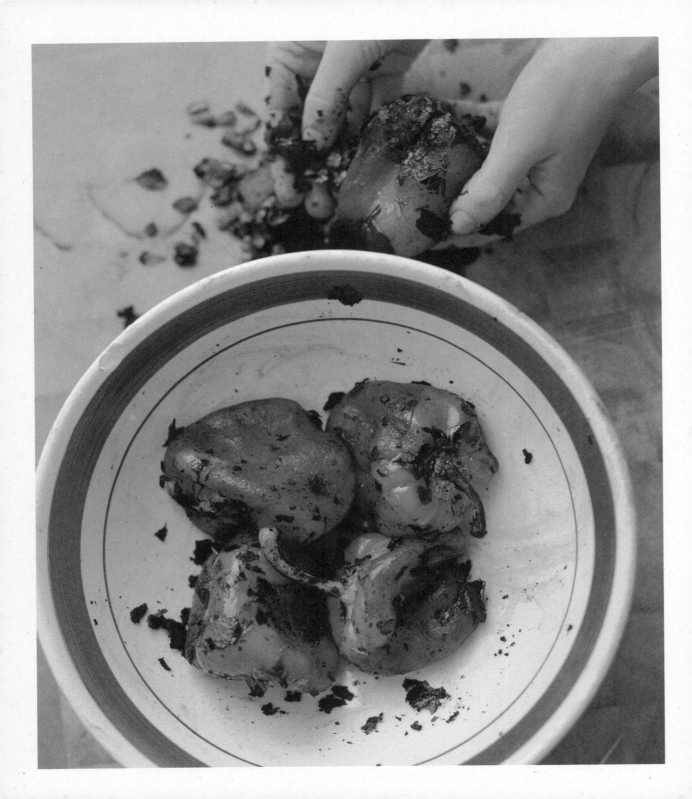

# Peppers

Ruby red. Sunshine yellow. Lava orange. Or just plain green.
Capsicum yourself silly.

## Charred peppers

If you don't have a griddle pan, here's a quick way to char peppers
on a gas burner. Turn your flame to medium and carefully place your
pepper over the flame, turning it round until it's black all over. Place in
a bowl, cover with clingfilm and leave to steam for a few minutes. Then
peel or wash off the blackened skin and use the sweet, smoky flesh to
chop into salads, pasta or whatever you like.

## Sweet roasted peppers

Cut 2 peppers in half, remove the seeds and pop into a roasting tin.
Add a few halved cherry tomatoes, some chopped black olives, some
torn-up basil and a drizzle of olive oil to each half, and roast in the
oven at 200°C/400°F/gas mark 6 for 45 minutes. Serve with brown
rice or couscous and a leafy salad for a super-quick tea.

## Slow-cooked peppers

Cut 2 red and 2 yellow peppers into long strips. Slowly cook in a pan
with a drizzle of olive oil and a peeled, crushed garlic clove over a
low heat for 20 minutes or so, until they are soft. Serve in a toasted
wholemeal pitta bread with some cream cheese for a snack, or on its
own as a side dish.

## Spicy roasted peppers

Cut 2 peppers in half, remove the seeds and pop into a roasting tin.
Add a tin of chopped tomatoes, a handful of raisins and a smaller
handful of toasted pine nuts, and sprinkle with a pinch each of ground
cinnamon and smoked paprika. Roast at 200°C/400°F/gas mark 6
for 45 minutes and serve with couscous and a leafy salad.

# Sweetcorn

**Little golden niblets of sweet sun-filled joy. Or kernels if you're being picky.**

### Spicy corn-on-the-cob

Bring a large pan of water to the boil. Add 4 corn on the cob, bring back to the boil, and cook for 8 to 10 minutes, until tender.

Meanwhile, finely chop 1 red chilli and mix with the juice of 1 lime, a knob of butter and a small handful of grated pecorino or Manchego cheese.

Once the corn is cooked, drain it in a colander. Then pop a corn holder or an old matchstick into both ends of each cob to act as handles. Serve on a plate with a generous spoonful of the spicy butter, and get rolling.

### Corn fritters

Strip the kernels off 2 cobs of corn, mix in a bowl with 1 tablespoon of self-raising flour, 1 egg and some finely chopped red chilli. Make little cakes out of the mixture and lightly fry in a little knob of butter. Serve with mashed avocado and some quick tomato salsa for a speedy lunch.

### Smoky corn

Cook 4 cobs of corn in boiling salted water for 5 minutes, then heat a griddle pan and grill until charred all over. Serve with lime wedges and a little knob of chilli butter.

### Crunchy corn

Toast some pumpkin seeds with a teaspoon of ground turmeric and cumin. Boil some sweetcorn kernels until tender, drain and return to the pan. Add the seeds and spices, stir well and serve with a spoonful of yoghurt.

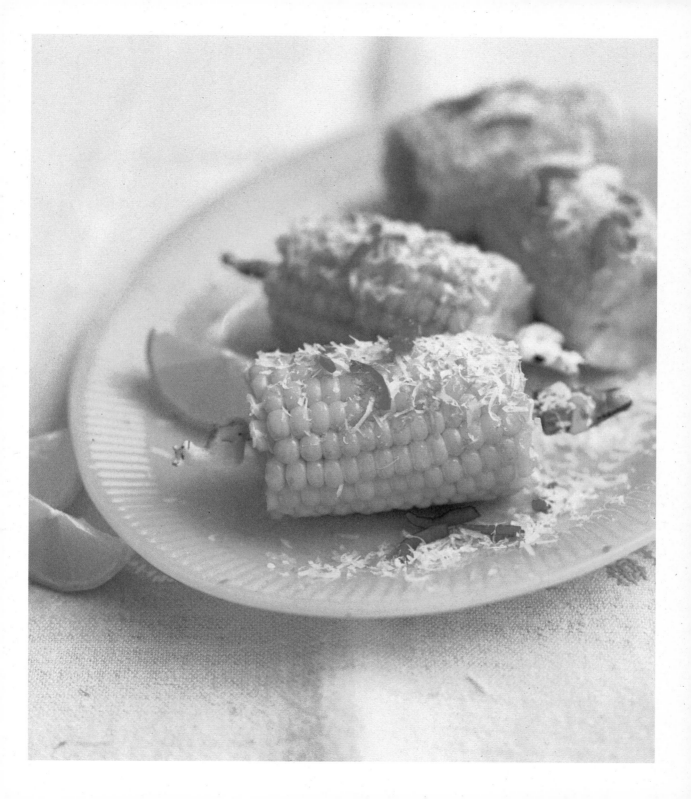

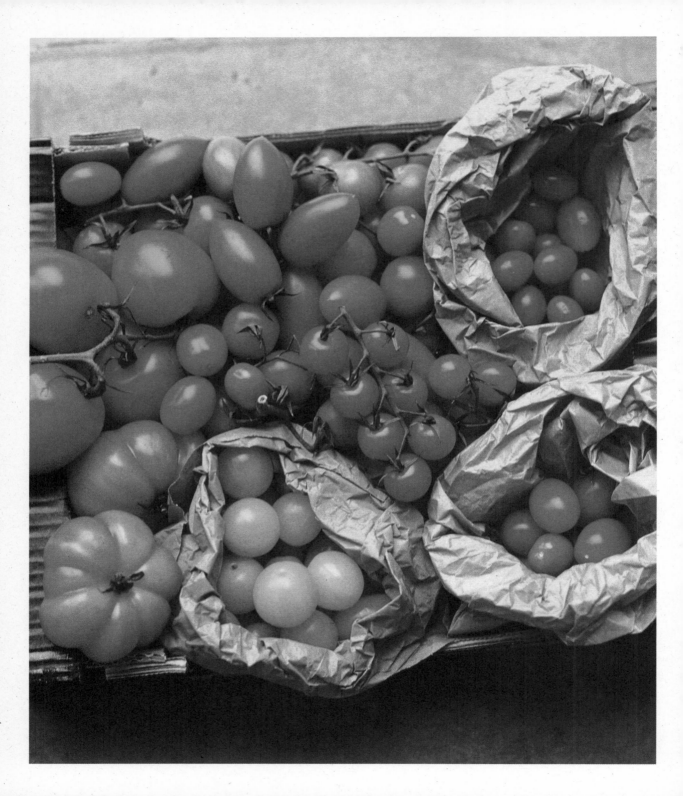

# Tomatoes

Pronounce their name however you like. They're still ace. Eat them in late summer if you want them at their very, very best.

### Roasted tomatoes

Mix several handfuls of cherry tomatoes with some peeled and sliced garlic cloves and a few sprigs of thyme and roast in the oven at 200°C/400°F/gas mark 6 for about 30 minutes. Serve squashed on to bread for lunch or breakfast, or as a side with dinner.

### Baked tomatoes

Cut the tops off 4 tomatoes and spoon out the centres. Drizzle some olive oil inside, sprinkle with salt, pepper and some thyme leaves, then pop a little knob of goat's cheese into each tomato. Bake at 180°C/350°F/gas mark 4 for 20 to 30 minutes, and serve with steamed rice or toasted flatbreads for a quick dinner.

### Indian spiced tomato salad

Toast 1 teaspoon of cumin seeds with 1 teaspoon of garam masala for a minute or so. Take off the heat and add a glug of oil to the pan. Mix well and then pour this over a bowl of 6 roughly chopped ripe tomatoes and a small handful of roughly chopped mint to serve.

### Tricolore salad

Slice a few tomatoes and put on a plate with slices of buffalo mozzarella, a drizzle of olive oil and some torn-up basil. Season well and serve as a light lunch or a side salad.

# GOOD THINGS TO HAVE FOR

# PUDDING

# Quick banana ice cream

Just plain yoghurt, a drizzle of honey and a couple of the yellow fellows that have gone a bit brown.

Serves 4
1 portion of your 5-a-day

4 ripe bananas
a generous squeeze of runny
   honey
seeds from 1 vanilla pod or
   1 teaspoon vanilla extract
1–2 tablespoons plain
   yoghurt

Peel the bananas, break them into chunks and pop them into the freezer. They need at least 2 hours, so it's good if you have a batch already in the freezer.

Make sure your food processor is set up with the normal blade, then put in all the ingredients and whizz until creamy.

Eat straight away or put into the freezer for an hour. After that, it'll go solid, so you'll have to wait for it to melt a bit.

Fancy a change? Try stirring in a handful of crushed meringue after blending for a crunchy ice cream.
Don't like bananas? Try replacing them with 4 big handfuls of frozen mixed berries instead.

# Monkeybockerglory

This dessert contains no old school pantaloons, maraschino cherries or organ-dancing simian types whatsoever. Fancy fan wafer optional.

Serves 4
counts towards your 5-a-day

**For the sundae**
1 lot of banana ice cream or
  8 scoops of good-quality
  vanilla ice cream
1 banana, chopped into
  rounds (or 4 handfuls of
  raspberries if you don't like
  bananas)
4 tablespoons crème fraîche

**For the chocolate sauce**
50g dark chocolate,
  broken up
50ml milk

**For the topping**
1 teaspoon of your favourite
  biscuit, crushed, or
  4 teaspoons of make-your-
  own muesli (page 58)

First make the chocolate sauce. Over a very low heat, melt the chocolate and the milk in a small pan. Once melted, turn up the heat, allow to simmer briefly, then immediately take off the heat.

Layer a couple of scoops of ice cream with the fruit in each bowl, add a blob of crème fraîche, drizzle with chocolate sauce and sprinkle with crushed biscuit or crunchy muesli.

# Fruit mess

**Pavlova suffered an architectural malfunction? Use any soft fruit you like (fresh berries, peaches and apricots in summer, or orchard fruits in winter) to recreate this healthier version of an Eton Mess.**

Serves 4
2½ portions of your 5-a-day

4 ripe pears, cored and cut into chunks
8 Victoria plums, stoned and cut into chunks
runny honey, for drizzling
a couple of handfuls of blackberries
8 tablespoons plain yoghurt or crème fraîche
1 teaspoon natural vanilla extract, or the seeds from 1 vanilla pod
1 good-quality shop-bought one-person meringue

Put the pears and plums into a pan with a squeeze of honey and a splash of water and simmer for a couple of minutes till slightly softened. Allow to cool, then stir in the blackberries.

Before serving, taste your fruit. If it makes you suck your cheeks in, add a little more honey and cook for another minute or so.

Mix the yoghurt or crème fraîche with another drizzle of honey and the vanilla.

Now get yourself 4 bowls and divide the fruit between them.

Top with the yoghurt and crumble over the meringue. Then get a spoon and mash it all together if you like.

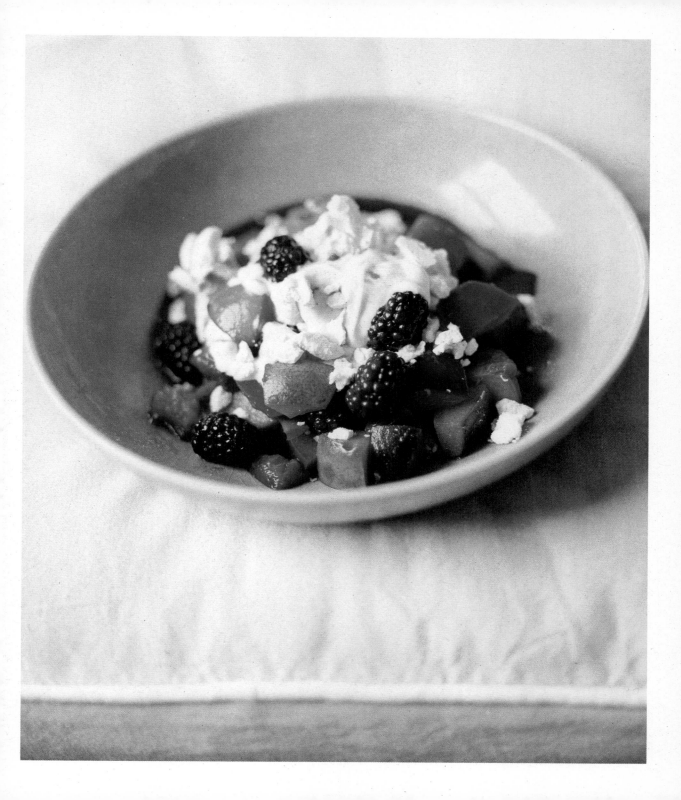

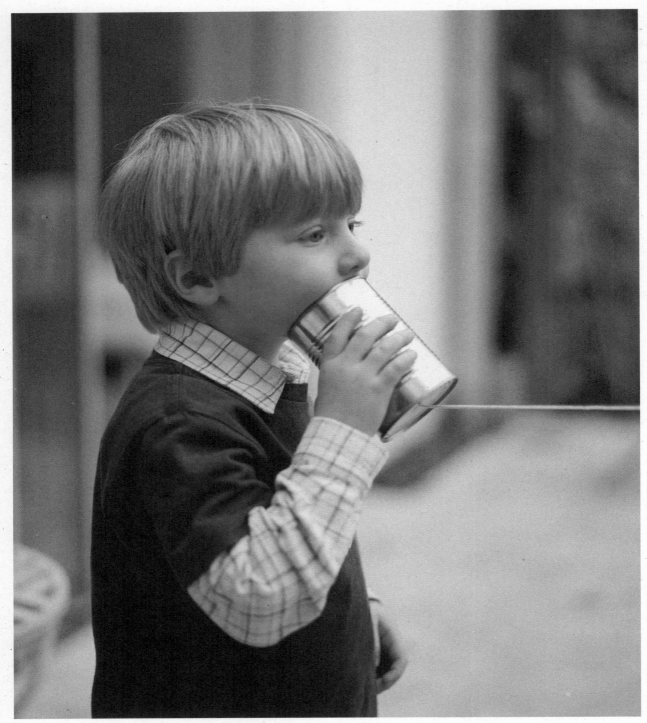

'Did you put mud in my sandwich?'

# Easy rice pud

The only easier version of this recipe is to eat your rice pudding plain. Which is decidedly less fun. You can use any fruit that's nearing the end of its days or is due to be sent to the Old Fruits' Home.*

Serves 4
1½ portions of your 5-a-day

2 x 400g tins of rice pudding
a few ginger nuts, smashed up in a sandwich bag
1 tablespoon muesli (shop-bought or make your own, see page 58)

For the compote
2 apples, cored and roughly chopped
2 pears, cored and roughly chopped
2 handfuls of fresh or frozen berries
2 tablespoons runny honey

To make the compote, put the fruit, honey and a splash of water into a little pan over a medium heat and allow to bubble away for 10 minutes, until the fruit has reduced down to a purée.

Heat your rice pudding in a pan until piping hot, then divide between 4 bowls. Swirl the fruit compote over the top and sprinkle with crushed ginger nuts and muesli.

*a.k.a. the compost heap

# Hot fruit

**We're talking about baked fruit here. Not the satsuma you nicked off the greengrocer or the grapes you're 'trialling' while pushing your trolley round the supermarket.**

Serves 4
1 portion of your 5-a-day

4 bananas, peeled
juice of 1 orange
juice of 1 lemon
runny honey, for drizzling
4 passion fruits, halved
2 limes, cut into wedges
4 tablespoons crème fraîche
    or plain yoghurt

Preheat your oven to 200°C/400°F/gas mark 6.

Tear off 4 big squares of foil. Lay a banana in the middle of each one, then fold the sides up a bit.

Squeeze the orange and lemon juice on to each piece of foil, followed by 1 teaspoon of honey, and fold each piece of foil over to make a parcel.

Bake in the oven for 15 minutes, then serve with the passion fruits (scoop out the pulp over your pudding), plus a squeeze of lime juice and a dollop of crème fraîche or yoghurt.

Not a fan of bananas?
Use 4 big apples with cores removed instead.

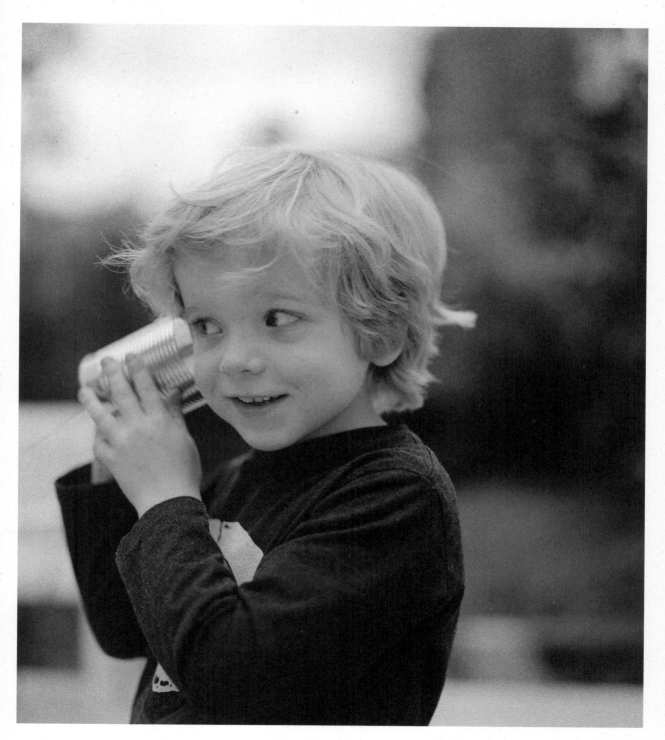

'Sorry, wrong number.'

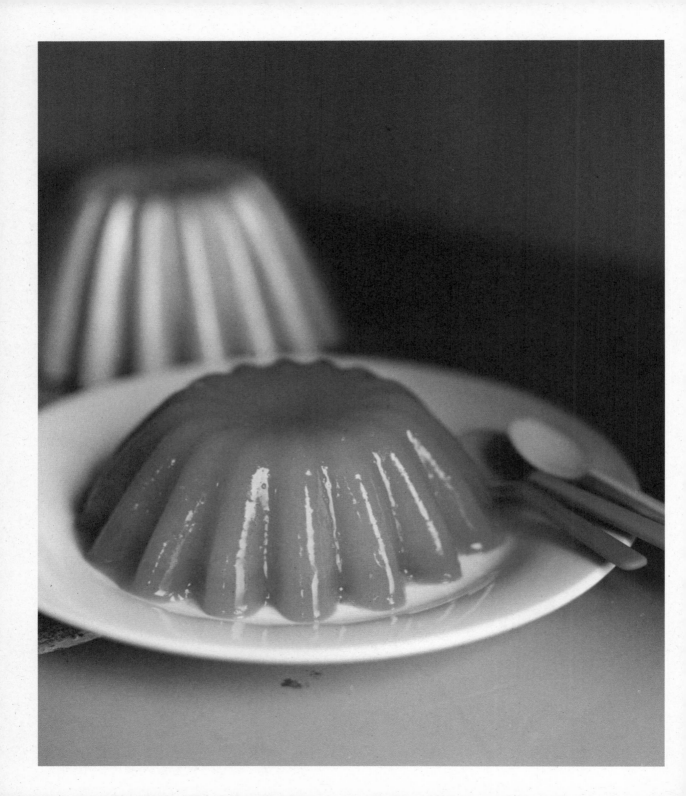

# Orange and strawberry jelly

## Wobble off.

Serves 4–6
1 portion of your 5-a-day

2 big handfuls of strawberries, stalks removed
juice of 6–8 big oranges (about 750ml juice)
juice of 1 lemon
100g golden caster sugar
7 small sheets of gelatine

Whizz two-thirds of the strawberries in a food processor. Put the mixture into a pan, add the orange and lemon juice and bring to the boil. Turn the heat off immediately, stir in the sugar until it has dissolved, then set aside to cool.

Lay the gelatine sheets side by side in a big bowl of cold water and leave to stand for 5 minutes.

Now pour the warm juice though a sieve into a jug. Remove the gelatine sheets from the water and add to the jug, stirring until fully dissolved.

Slice the remaining strawberries into a clear serving bowl or 4–6 individual glasses. Pour the jelly mix over them, cover with an upturned plate or some clingfilm, then put into the fridge and leave to set for at least 4 hours.

Once set, serve the jelly either on its own or with a generous scoop of vanilla ice cream or a blob of crème fraîche.

Feel free to add more whole fruit to your jelly. Sliced peaches, raspberries and peeled clementine segments all work really well.

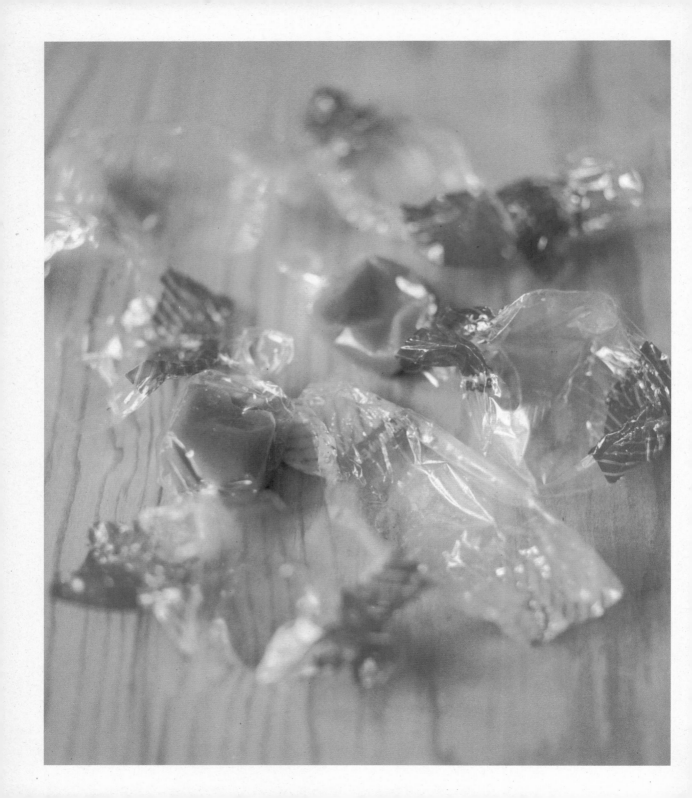

# Sticky toffee pudding

Six of the tastiest syllables in the English language, this pudding is as good as it sounds. And soaking the dates in coffee gives it a rich malty flavour without making the pudding taste of old espresso. Clever.

Serves 4–6
counts towards your 5-a-day

**For the pudding**
150g stoned dates, finely chopped
1 teaspoon bicarbonate of soda
1 shot of strong espresso, or 4 teaspoons instant coffee made up with a little water
250ml boiling water
50g unsalted butter, at room temperature
100g golden caster sugar
2 large free-range eggs, beaten
150g self-raising flour
a pinch of ground cinnamon
a pinch of grated nutmeg

**For the toffee sauce**
50g butter
100g soft brown sugar
1 vanilla pod
75ml double cream
a big handful of toasted pecans, roughly chopped (optional)

Preheat your oven to 180°C/350°F/gas mark 4.

Put the chopped dates, bicarbonate of soda and coffee into a bowl and cover with the boiling water. Leave to soak for 10 minutes while you get on with the rest of the pudding.

In a second bowl, beat together the butter and sugar until pale and fluffy. Stir in the eggs, flour and spices and mix well.

After the dates have had 10 minutes of soaking, drain them and stir them into the pudding mixture.

Butter a medium-sized ovenproof dish, pour in the mixture and bake for 30 to 40 minutes, until golden brown.

Meanwhile, make the sauce. Put all the sauce ingredients (apart from the nuts) into a pan and melt over a low heat until you have a smooth, rich toffee sauce. You can stir in the toasted pecans now, if using.

Once the pudding is cooked, serve it in generous scoops, drizzled with the toffee sauce, and with a blob of crème fraîche alongside.

You can make this in individual ramekins if you like. The pudding freezes beautifully either way, in one dish or in ramekins.

# Quick St Clement's trifle

Oranges, lemons and some old coins aside, this trifle can be put together in under 10 minutes. No trifling around whatsoever. Feel free to add a splash of limoncello if you want to liven things up for the grown-ups.

Serves 4–6

200g shop-bought Madeira cake, cut into thick slices

zest and juice of 1 lemon

zest and juice of 1 orange

limoncello (optional)

200g lemon curd

500ml custard (tinned is best as it sets thicker than the posh runny stuff)

300ml double cream

2 tablespoons golden caster sugar

seeds from 1 vanilla pod

Layer the bottom of your fanciest dish with the slices of cake.

Finely grate the zest of the lemon and the orange into a bowl and put to one side for later. Cut the lemon and orange in half and squeeze the juice over the cake. If you want to add some booze, splash or douse the cake in limoncello.

Spread the lemon curd over the cake. Then pour over the custard and put in the fridge for the flavours to mingle while you whip the cream.

Put the cream, sugar and vanilla seeds into a bowl and whisk away until the cream forms soft peaks.

Pile the cream on top of the custard, using a spoon to create little peaks. Sprinkle with the citrus zest.

You can make this in individual bowls if you've got a bit more time.

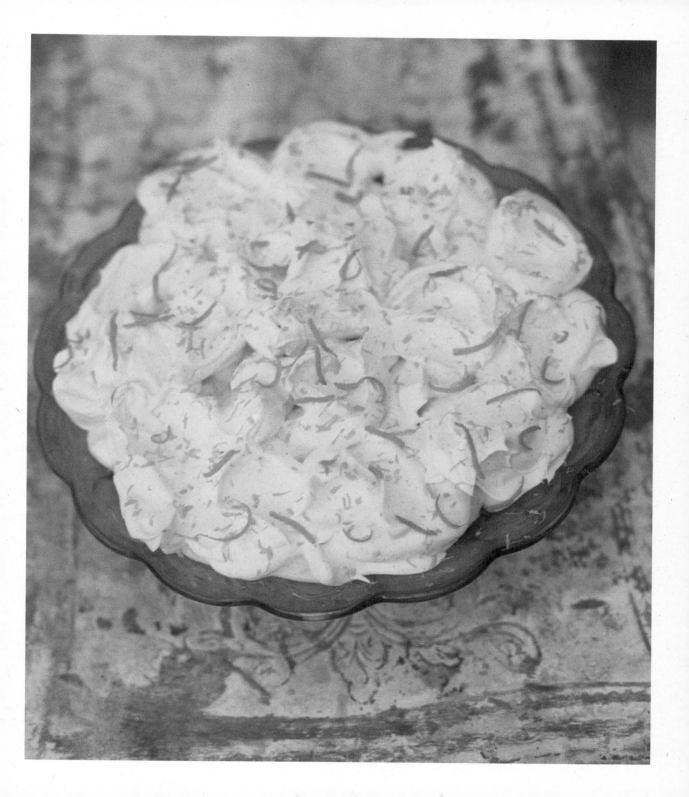

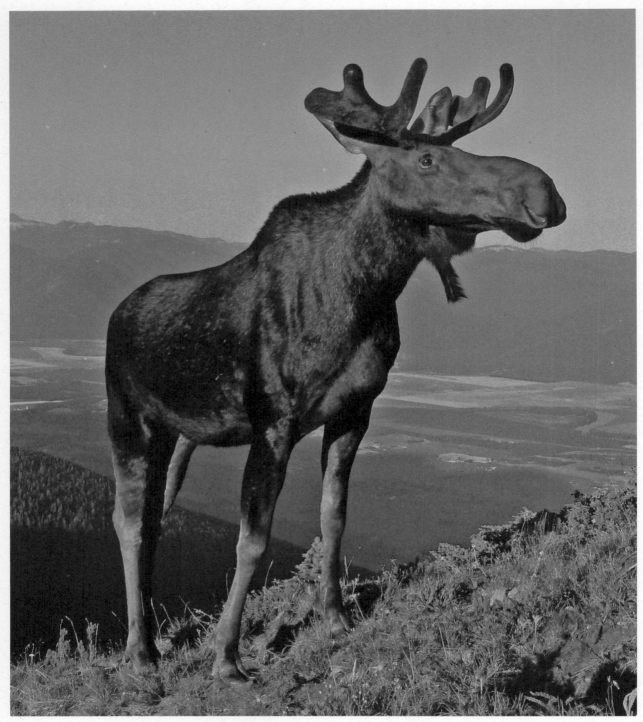

'I'm kind of brown and I'm a moose. Deal with it.'

# Chocolate mousse with sticky orange caramel

All hail the inventor of mousse, who was planning to make a cake but got sidetracked listening to a radio programme about nutmeg, forgot to add the flour and ended up with sweet, fluffy soup.

Serves 4

For the mousse
200g good-quality dark chocolate
4 large free-range eggs (2 yolks; 4 whites)
50g golden caster sugar
a tiny pinch of salt

For the caramel
150ml orange juice
150g golden caster sugar

Break up the chocolate and put it into a heatproof glass bowl. Boil a small pan of water, then turn down the heat, prop the glass bowl above it so that the bowl doesn't touch the water. Allow the chocolate to melt, resisting the temptation to stir or eat it all.

Once melted, take the chocolate off the heat and set it aside to cool.

Separate the eggs. Whisk the egg whites with half the sugar until they form soft peaks.

Then stir 2 yolks, the rest of the sugar and the pinch of salt into the cooled chocolate and slowly mix together. Save the extra yolks for an omelette or making your own custard.

Once mixed, gently fold in the foamy egg whites. Pour the mousse into a serving bowl and pop it into the fridge for about 30 minutes.

Make the caramel just before you're about to eat. Heat the orange juice and sugar in a pan on a low heat, and simmer for 5 minutes, until the edges start to brown. Keep stirring until the sauce turns a deep orangey brown.

Add 50ml water, keep stirring, and cook for another couple of minutes. Then pour the caramel into a bowl and leave in the fridge to cool down a little.

Serve big dollops of mousse drizzled with orange caramel, with a blob of crème fraîche.

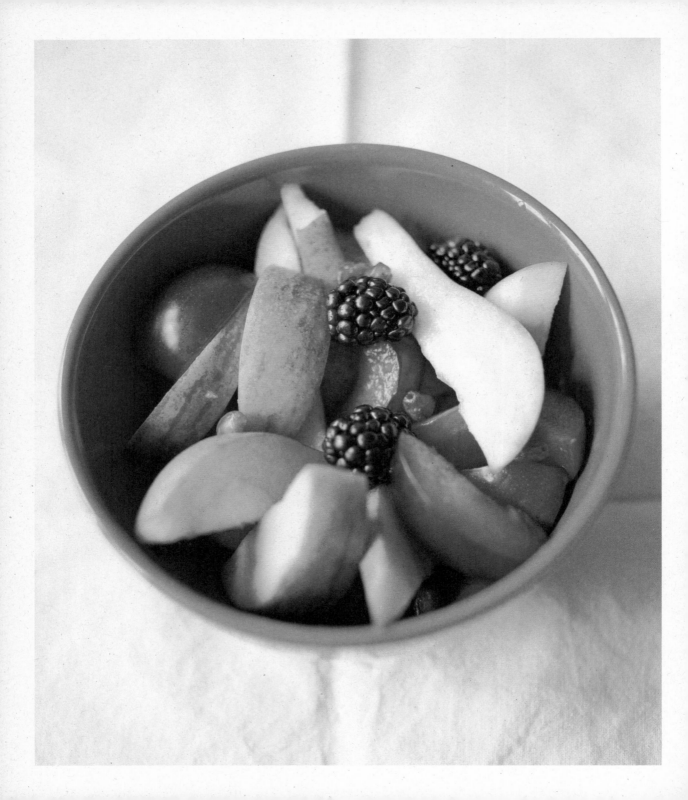

# QUICK THINGS TO DO WITH

---

# FRUIT

Here's a small wheelbarrow full of simple tasty tricks to increase your daily fruit intake and make pudding even more exciting.

Try popping your oranges in the fridge as this helps them keep longer and makes them taste super refreshing.

Make your own fruit kebabs by chopping up a mixture of your favourite seasonal fruits, skewering them onto wooden kebab sticks, drizzling with a little bit of honey and popping them under the grill for a couple of minutes.

Freezing grapes turns them into instant mini ice lollies.

Or if these aren't enough to get you dancing merrily round the fruit bowl, why not have a go at some of the ideas over the page ...

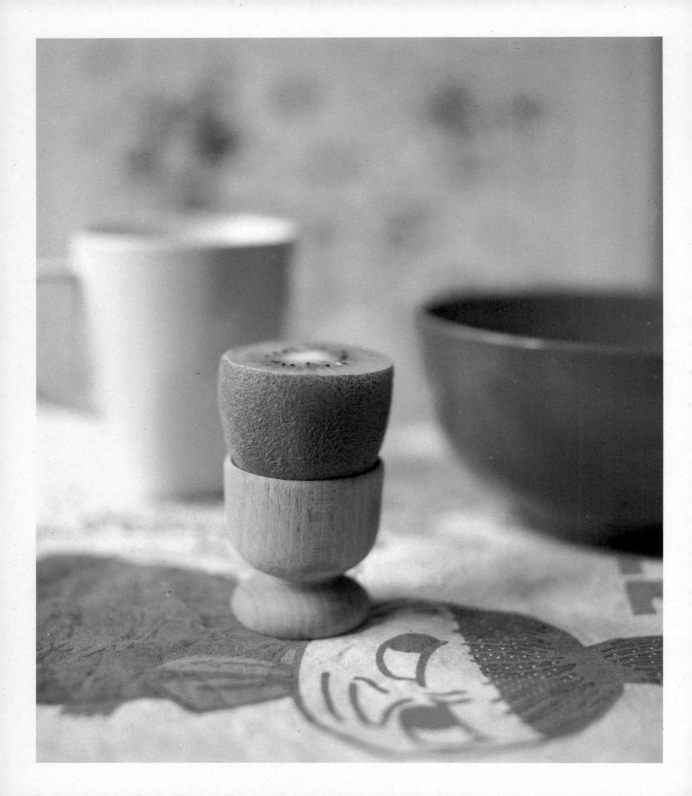

Summer fruit salad: Stone a punnet of cherries, 2 peaches or nectarines, then chop with a punnet of strawberries and give everything a good rinse. Peel and chop 1 mango and ½ pineapple. Mix it all together in a bowl with a splash of smoothie or orange juice. Serves 4 and is 2½ portions of your 5-a-day.

Autumn fruit salad: Core 2 apples and 4 pears, stone 4 plums and chop them all up together. Put in a bowl and, using your hands, squash a handful of blackberries over the top. Make a hole in the top of a pomegranate and squeeze the juice out on to the salad. Remove the 'jewels' from inside the pomegranate and sprinkle over the top. Serves 4 and is 1½ portions of your 5-a-day.

Apple and cheese: Slice up some apples, cut some Cheddar cheese into chunks and pop on to a little plate with some oatcakes.

Grated apples and pears: Grate up an apple or pear, stir into plain yoghurt with some ground cinnamon and a little drizzle of honey for a grate pud (sorry). Try adding a handful of raisins or chopped dried apricots.

Blindfold taste test: Chop up lots of different fruit, then take it in turns to wear a blindfold and see who can guess the most fruit, just by taste.

Spin the bottle: Place a selection of fruit (apple slices, clementine segments, berries) in a circle on a clean surface, mixed in with nuts and a few pieces of chocolate. Pop an empty bottle in the middle and spin to see who gets what.

Quick chocolate fondue: Break 50g chocolate into a glass, heatproof bowl, add a splash of milk or water, and pop over a pan of boiling water. Once melted, pour into a little bowl and dip in chopped-up fruit.

Green eggs: Cut a kiwi in half, pop it into an eggcup, add a teaspoon and give thanks to the hairy chicken.

# Harrison
## and the
# prawns

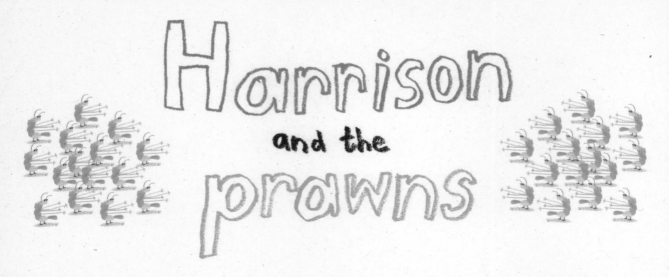

'Harrison? Are you in bed?' his Dad called from downstairs. 'Just cleaning my teeth, Dad,' shouted Harrison. Harrison had been cleaning his teeth for quite a long time now, not because he liked cleaning his teeth but because he didn't like going to bed. Going to bed and going to sleep? Thought Harrison. How boring is that?

'Come on,' said his Mum, coming up the stairs, 'time for bed.' 'But I don't want to go to bed,' he said. 'It's boring.' 'Going to bed might be boring but going to sleep is brilliant,' said his Mum. 'What do you mean?' said Harrison. 'Because when you go to sleep you can dream and dreams can be the most exciting things ever.' 'Really? Do you think?' said Harrison and he put his toothbrush in the cup and went off to his room to bed. 'Night night,' said his Mum. 'Night night,' said Harrison. He closed his eyes and soon he was asleep and not long after that he began to dream.

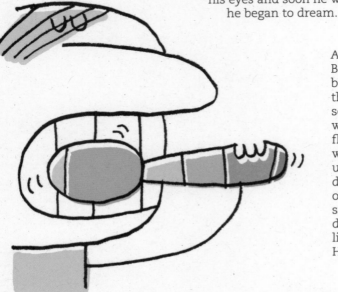

At first all he could see were clouds. Big fluffy white clouds. Not in the sky, but right in front of his nose. Then they began to clear and Harrison could see a field of flowers. Flowers that lay wilting and miserable. 'Those poor flowers,' said Harrison, 'I wonder what's wrong with them.' He looked up and next to them lay a big, lazy dragon snoozing in the sun. Every so often the dragon would do a big, smelly trump and the flowers would droop and wilt some more. 'I wouldn't like to be one of those flowers,' said Harrison. 'That dragon needs to move.'

'Absolutely,' said a toothbrush stood next to him. 'But how do we do it, Harrison?' Harrison had never met a talking toothbrush before but he seemed to recognise it from somewhere. 'Are you my toothbrush?' said Harrison, 'From the bathroom?' 'Yes I am,' said the toothbrush. 'What are you doing here?' 'Well, I suppose you spent so long cleaning your teeth tonight I must have stayed in your memory and now I'm here in your dream.' 'You mean if I think about something when I'm awake, it could appear in my dreams?' 'Correct,' answered the toothbrush. 'Well,' said Harrison, 'it's nice to meet you, I mean I suppose I've met you before but I've never spoken to you.' 'The pleasure's all mine,' said the toothbrush. 'Now, what are we going to do about this pesky dragon?'

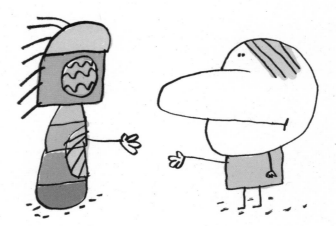

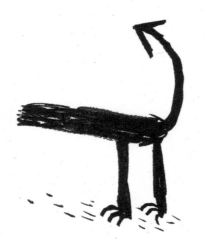

'Well, I suppose we better go and see if we can get him to move,' replied Harrison. 'Good idea,' said the toothbrush, so they went over and stood at the dragon's feet. Harrison called up to him. 'Excuse me! Mr Dragon?' But the dragon couldn't hear him. 'I say, dragon, old bean, you wouldn't mind shifting would you?' shouted the toothbrush but the dragon did not respond. 'If only there was a way of getting closer to his ears,' said Harrison. 'Absolutely,' said the toothbrush. 'But they're just so very high up.'

The next day Harrison woke up and his dream had ended but all he could think about was the dragon. How could he get closer to his ears? How would you get closer to a dragon's ears? Harrison got out of bed, went into the bathroom and cleaned his teeth. Suddenly he had an idea.

He rushed downstairs into the kitchen. 'Mum! Mum! Have we got any tin foil?' 'Yes, I think so,' said his Mum. 'In the bottom drawer, what do want tin foil for?' 'To wrap around my feet, of course,' said Harrison. He pulled off two big sheets of tin foil and wrapped them round each of his feet. He wore the tin foil all day until bedtime and, for once, he couldn't wait to go to bed. He brushed his teeth and climbed into bed. He closed his eyes and soon he was asleep and not long after that he began to dream.

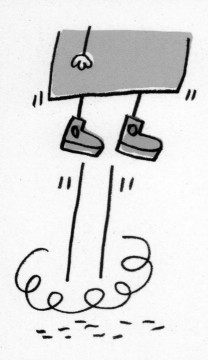

The white clouds parted and the dragon was still there, laying in the sun, still doing enormous trumps on all the flowers. 'Hello there, Harrison,' said the toothbrush. 'Had any ideas about how we're going to shift this smelly creature?' Harrison looked down at his feet and his plan had worked! He was now wearing a shiny pair of rocket boots. 'Golly!' said the toothbrush. 'Look at those!' Harrison pushed the big red button that said 'PUSH' and he shot into the sky. He pointed his arms towards the dragon's head and within seconds he was hovering right next to the dragon's ears.

'Excuse me?' shouted Harrison. The dragon looked at him. 'What do you want?' 'I'd like you to move out of the way, you're damaging these flowers.' 'I shall do no such thing,' said the dragon, 'I'm going nowhere.' 'But you can go anywhere you want to, these flowers can't move!' pleaded Harrison. 'I couldn't care less,' said the dragon. 'Now go away.' If only there was a way of getting him to move, thought Harrison. How on earth will I do that?

Harrison woke up the next day. He lay in bed desperately thinking of what to do. What would you do, if you had to try and move a great, big dragon? He looked at all the things in his bedroom. He looked at his cuddly owl, he looked at his toy planes, he looked at his tool set. He couldn't think of anything. He went into his little sister's room and looked at her toys. A kitchen, a teddy bear, an umbrella. None of these would do either.

He went downstairs and walked into the kitchen 'What do you want, more tin foil?' said his Mum, smiling. 'Not this time, Mum,' said Harrison, 'Tin foil won't work.' 'What's in the fridge, Mum?' he asked. 'Have a look,' said his Mum. He opened the fridge and had a good look around. Milk? No. Yoghurt? No. Cheese? No. Prawns? Prawns? Prawns.

'Mum, what are you doing with these prawns?' 'I was going to cook them for dinner,' said his Mum. 'Could I help you cook dinner?' said Harrison. 'Yes, you can help,' said his Mum. That night as they prepared dinner Harrison stared at the prawns and as they went into the hot pan he continued to stare at them and as his family ate them for dinner he stared at them some more. As soon as he had finished dinner Harrison asked if he could go to bed. 'Bed?' said his Dad. 'Are you okay? You never normally want to go to bed.' 'I've got things to do Dad,' said Harrison. 'Busy night ahead.' He ran upstairs, put on his pyjamas, cleaned his teeth and got into bed. He closed his eyes and soon he was asleep and not long after that he began to dream.

The white clouds parted and there lay the lazy dragon, trumping away. 'Got to say, I thought those rocket boots would have worked last night,' said the toothbrush. 'What's the plan now?' 'Come with me,' said Harrison. They walked over to the dragon and he looked right down his huge nose at them. 'If you think you're moving me, you've got another thing coming,' he sneered and did another great big trump. 'That's what you think,' said Harrison. 'I'm going to to make you move whether you like it or not.' 'Ha! You and whose army?' laughed the dragon. 'This army,' said a prawn. A prawn wearing a helmet.

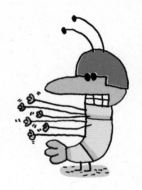

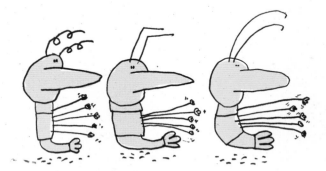

'Yes, this army,' said another prawn standing behind him, also wearing a helmet. Harrison turned around and there stood a humungous army of prawns, all wearing helmets, all standing to attention. 'Huh, how are a lot of little prawns, a little boy and a silly toothbrush going to move a dragon as big as me?' 'I'll show you how,' said Harrison. 'Ready prawns?' 'Ready!' they all shouted. 'Go!'

The prawns raced forward and buried themselves beneath the dragon's body. They then started to tickle him. They tickled and tickled and tickled him and the dragon started to smile and then he started to laugh. He laughed and he laughed until tears rolled down his face. He began to wriggle and squirm and he stood up on his back legs as he couldn't take the tickling any longer and he ran away, far away, trumping as he went. The flowers lifted their heads and stood tall for the first time in weeks. They breathed in the fresh air and bathed in the warm sunlight. 'We did it!' said Harrison. 'Jolly well done everybody,' said the toothbrush.

The next evening, just before bedtime, Harrison went and found his Mum in the sitting room. He had something important to tell her. 'What is it Harrison?' asked his Mum. 'Mum. You know what? I've been thinking. You were right. Going to bed might not be a lot of fun but going to sleep can be the most exciting thing you do all day.'

And off he went, up the stairs.

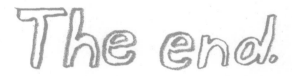
The end.

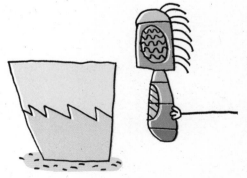

# GOOD THINGS TO

---

# MAKE
# AND
# BAKE

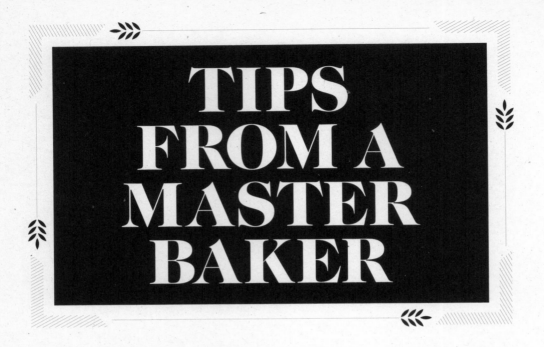

# TIPS FROM A MASTER BAKER

When it comes to bread, what Andrew Whitley doesn't know about baking isn't worth knowing. Having set up The Village Bakery, Melmerby in 1976, Andrew now teaches breadmaking, campaigns for better food and farming, and has written his own book *Bread Matters* (Fourth Estate, 2006).

He's also behind the 'Real Bread Campaign' (www.breadmatters.com), which aims to bring real bread back to our kitchens and shelves and 'Bake your Lawn', geared specifically towards getting children involved in breadmaking, from seed to sandwich. Here are his top 10 tips to baking better bread.

### 1. TAKE YOUR TIME

Fast bread bad, slow bread good. Using too much yeast or making too warm a dough leads to crumbly bread that dries out quickly. Start the night before if you can, and make a sponge (flour, water and yeast). Then add the rest of the ingredients (flour, water, salt and any seeds, herbs or spices) in the morning for better taste and better texture.

### 2. LONGER EQUALS FRESHER

The longer you give your bread to rise, the longer it will stay fresh after baking. More nutrients (like folate acid) get released, making it more nourishing and easier to digest. Bread made too fast doesn't release nutrients properly, which can lead to indigestion and bloating.

### 3. KNEAD WATER, NOT FLOUR

When kneading, use water instead of extra flour if your dough starts sticking. Keep a bowl nearby and moisten your hands and work surface with a little water. Adding more flour just makes for tighter, drier, brick-like loaves.

## 4. THE WETTER, THE BETTER

Within reason, the wetter your dough is, the better the eating quality of your bread will be.
A soft, moist dough, even if it's a bit sticky on the surface, will rise much better.

## 5. BREAD LIKES TO RISE IN A DRAUGHT FREE, SLIGHTLY HUMID SPOT

Leaving your dough by a radiator or covering it with a damp tea towel are rubbish tips. Instead, pop your loaf tin into a big carrier bag, tape up any holes, blow the bag up like a balloon and tie up the ends to keep the warm air in. That way, the bag won't stick to the dough and it'll expand nicely without drying out.

## 6. PUSHED FOR TIME? NO NEED TO KNEAD

You can make bread without kneading at all. Just reduce the yeast to about 10% of what the recipe says, mix all the ingredients together until a dough is formed, put it into a tin and allow to rise for at least 12 hours. Perfect for making in the evening and then baking first thing in the morning.

## 7. OLD DOUGH MAKES FOR TASTIER NEW DOUGH

For tastier, longer lasting bread, keep a lump of dough from the loaf you're making and use it the next time you're baking. Old dough keeps in the fridge for about a week (it's okay if it goes a bit sludgy). The old dough should be no more than 10% of the total amount of dough you're baking. The science reason for this is that as dough ferments, it generates acid and acidity makes for a more rounded bready flavour.

## 8. A MESSY BAKER COVERS THEIR TRACKS

Shaping issues? Raggedy looking bread? Try dipping the top into flour, sesame or poppy seeds or oat flakes first. It makes your bread look more rustic and attractive whilst covering up hurried workmanship.

## 9. WASH UP IN COLD WATER

This is the only time you break the 10 commandments of washing up. If you wash up doughy bowls and utensils in hot water, the starch in the dough becomes gelatinised by the heat. Which makes everything more sticky and even more difficult to scrub off.

## 10. SOAK THE EXTRAS

If you're planning on adding seeds, nuts or dried fruit to your bread, try soaking them in a little water or fruit juice first. Otherwise they'll rob moisture from the dough and make for dry bread. So, if you're adding 200g of fruit and nuts, soak them in up to 40ml or 20% of liquid. Put everything into a polythene bag, swirl it around and leave for a few hours. Then drain off any excess liquid before adding to your dough.

### (AN EXTRA BOOZY TIP)

For even better bread, before you pop your empty real ale or wine bottles in the recycling,
swill out the dregs with a little water and add to your dough. The alcohol gets burnt off during
baking, so no need to worry about boozy bread.

# Tomato and thyme focaccia

The original tear-and-share bread. Once baked, place on the table, take a corner each, count to three and tug for dear life.

Makes one 20 x 35cm focaccia
counts towards your 5-a-day

1 x 7g sachet of dried quick-action yeast
1 teaspoon runny honey
500g strong white bread flour
a pinch of salt
2 handfuls of cherry tomatoes
2 garlic cloves, peeled and sliced
a small bunch of thyme, stalks removed
olive oil

First measure out 250ml tepid water. Tepid means it should be the same temperature as your body. In other words, you should be able to stick your finger in it without crying. Too hot will kill the yeast, too cold won't get it working.

Add the yeast and honey to the water and wait for it to bubble. Meanwhile, put your flour in a big mixing bowl and make a well in the middle. Add the salt to the bubbling yeast mixture, then pour it into the middle of the flour and use a fork to bring it together.

Once it has come together, knead it into a ball. It should be a bit wetter than the average bread dough so add more water if needed.

Next, place it on a clean work surface and knead away for 5 minutes or so, until you have a super-smooth elastic dough. Pop inside a big plastic bag and follow tip 5 on page 281. Then leave to rise for 40 minutes.

Meanwhile, squash the tomatoes into a bowl with your hands. Add the garlic, thyme leaves and a little olive oil and mix together.

Once the dough has risen, put it on to an oiled 20 x 35cm baking tray, using your hands to gently stretch and pull it to the shape of the tray. Pop it back in the plastic bag again and leave to rise for another 30 to 40 minutes.

Drain any excess juicy stuff from the tomato mixture and scatter the mixture over the dough. Dip your fingers in some flour and poke holes in the dough, then leave to rise again for a final 40 minutes. While this is happening, preheat your oven to 220°C/425°F/gas mark 7.

Bake the focaccia for 30 to 40 minutes, until puffed up and golden.

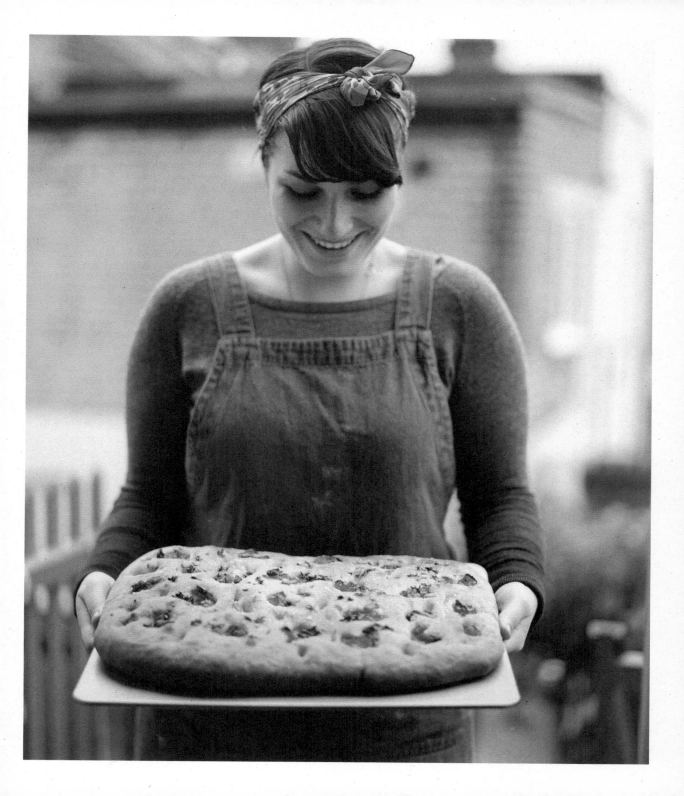

# Half and half bread

Half white, half brown, wholly fulfilling. This loaf is perfect for the indecisive, those trying to convert diehard white bread fans and everyone else who knows which side their bread is buttered. Also a great place to start if you've never baked bread before.

Makes 1 decent loaf
250g white bread flour
250g brown bread flour
1 x 7g sachet of dried quick-
    action yeast
1 teaspoon sea salt

Measure out 350ml tepid water (you should be able to stick a finger in it without yelping). Mix the flours, yeast and salt together in a bowl and stir in the water until you have a big pasty mess. Pop the bowl in a big plastic bag and follow tip 5 on page 281. Then leave for a few minutes to allow the yeast to start working.

After a couple of minutes, take the dough out of the bowl and knead on a clean surface until it becomes smooth. Put it back into the bowl, pop it back in the bag again and leave to rise for an hour or so. By the time you come back, it should have doubled in size.

After an hour, take the dough out of the bowl, knead for 30 seconds, then shape it into a flat oval. Put it on to a baking tray and put it back into the plastic bag again to rise for 40 minutes or so.

Preheat your oven to 220°C/425°F/gas mark 7. When the dough has had its 40 minutes, slash the top a few times with a knife and dust with a little flour. Half fill another baking tray with water and place on the bottom of your oven. This will create steam as the loaf bakes and help give your bread a lovely crust and texture.

Bake the loaf in the oven for 35 to 40 minutes, until golden. To check if your bread is ready, lift up the loaf and give it a tap on the bottom. If it sounds hollow like a drum, it's good.

# howies DohBOY
*a simple lad.*

In the beginning, bread was simple. Flour. Water. Yeast. A little salt. And plenty of that most important ingredient: time. The staff of life, they used to call it. Then things got a bit more complicated. In 1961, they found a faster way. The Chorleywood Way. More yeast. And a new ingredient: fat. Fat increased the shelf life, sponginess and, of course, profits. Good for those making it. Not so good for those eating it.

So please say hello to Doh Boy. Created by the good folk over at howies, his mission is to take the fat and all the other weird stuff out of bread. After all, we don't knead it. The only reason it's there is to help make bread bake quicker and keep it on the shelf for longer. Doh Boy thinks the Chorleywood technique has made fatter profits for those who make and sell it. But it has also made us all a little fatter as a result.

You expect there to be fat in a chocolate bar. But you don't expect it in your daily bread.

Doh Boy is leading the fight for a return to simple. To good old-fashioned bread that not only tastes of something, but contains no rubbish whatsoever. So make like Doh Boy and bake your own.

howies®

# Cheese twigs

Officially known as grissini, betterly known as cheese twigs, these DIY breadsticks are really easy to make. Great for snacks, crumbling into soups and serving at posh cocktail parties.

Makes lots
300g plain flour
1 teaspoon sea salt
1 x 7g sachet of dried quick-
    action yeast
75g unsalted butter
75g Cheddar cheese, grated
150ml warm milk

Put the flour, salt and yeast into a bowl. In the same way you'd make a crumble, rub the butter into the flour with your fingers until you have fine breadcrumbs. Add the grated cheese and mix in well.

Next, pour in the warm milk and mix with a fork until you have a soft and sticky dough. Cover the bowl with a plastic bag as in tip 5 on page 281 and leave to prove for an hour.

After an hour, take the dough out, give it a quick knead, then pop it back into the bowl, cover with the bag again and leave for another 30 minutes.

Preheat your oven to 150°C/300°F/gas mark 2.

After the dough has had its 30 minutes, use a rolling pin to roll it out to 1cm thick, trying not to use any flour. Cut the dough into strips and roll each one between your hands into a long pencil shape.

Lay them on a greaseproof-lined tray and bake in the oven for 20 to 25 minutes. Allow to cool and store in an airtight container for up to a week.

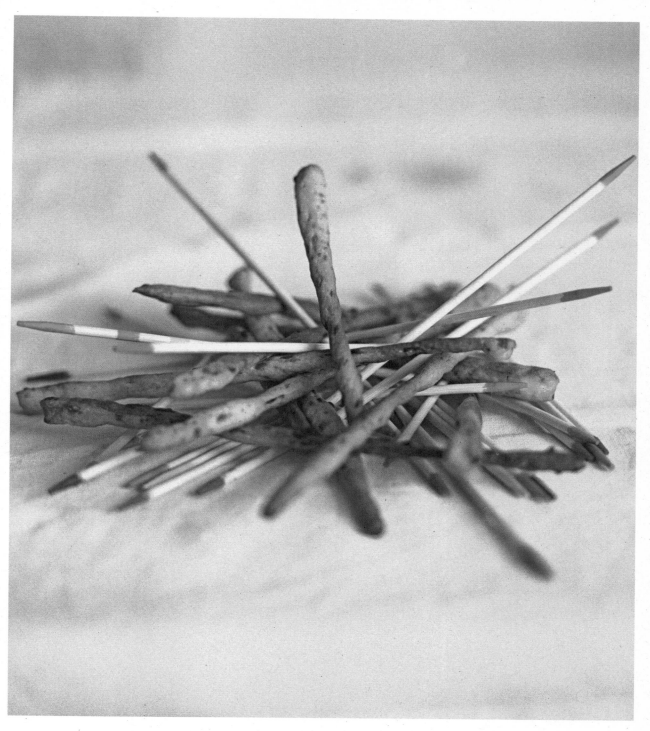

Pick-up-twigs. Before everyone else does.

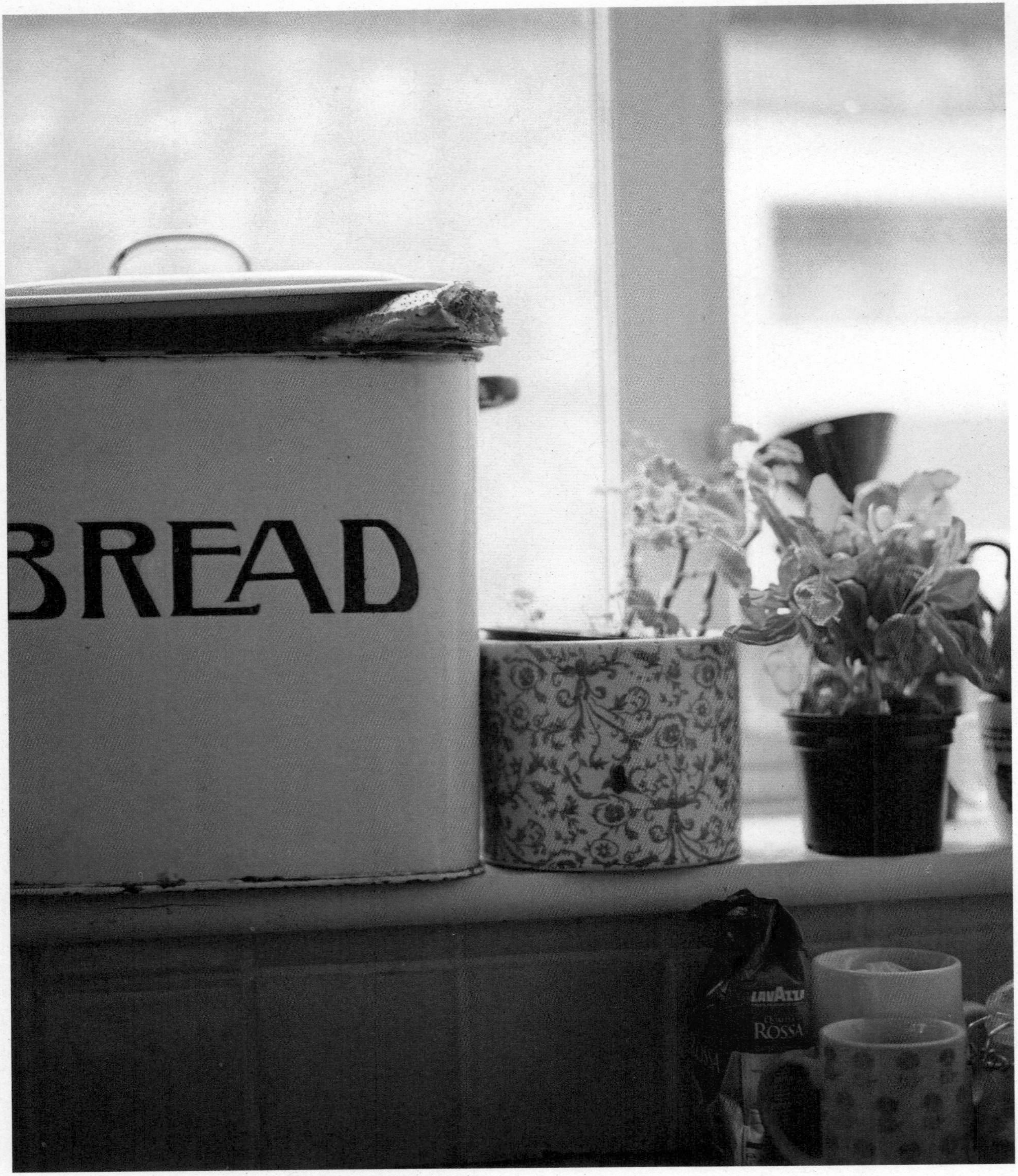
BREAD
ROSSA

# Secret sausage rolls

Apple, apricot, red onion – they're all hidden inside these crispy little rolls. Counting towards your 5-a-day, they're far better than the flabby high-street versions and brilliant for lunchboxes, picnics and parties.

Makes 12 sausage rolls
counts towards your 5-a-day

olive oil
1 red onion, peeled and finely chopped
1 eating apple, cored and finely chopped
a few sprigs of thyme, stalks removed
freshly grated nutmeg
a small handful of dried apricots, finely chopped
6 good-quality pork sausages
plain flour, for dusting
1 pack of best-quality shop-bought puff pastry
1 large free-range egg
a splash of milk
a little handful of sesame or poppy seeds

Preheat your oven to 190°C/375°F/gas mark 5 and line a baking tray with greaseproof paper.

Heat a splash of olive oil in a frying pan and cook the chopped onion over a medium heat until soft. Add the chopped apple and the thyme leaves and cook for another couple of minutes.

Place in a bowl to cool, then add the grated nutmeg and chopped apricots. Squeeze the sausages out of their skins and into the bowl, and mush the whole lot up with your hands. Set aside.

Dust a clean work surface with flour and roll out the puff pastry to the thickness of a pound coin and the size of an A4 piece of paper. Cut it down the middle into 2 long rectangles.

Lay the sausage mixture in 2 lines just off centre of the pastry rectangles, making sure to leave a 2cm border either side. Beat the egg and milk together in a bowl.

Using a pastry brush, brush down the long edge of each rectangle with the egg mix and then fold the pastry over to wrap up the sausage mixture. Use a fork to seal the long edges together and cut each one into 4cm chunky rolls.

Brush the rolls with the egg mixture, sprinkle with seeds and place on the prepared baking tray. Bake in the oven for 20 to 25 minutes, until golden brown. Either eat while still warm or allow to cool, wrap in foil and pop into tomorrow's lunchbox.

# A Guide to Nicking Stuff

## HUNGRY?

Strapped for cash? Sofa too far from the shop? Been told you can't eat that pie?

Here's how to eat for nothing without leaving the house....

Being HOME ALONE helps

NEVER EVER finish the milk → it's just not worth it.

And look out for milk moustaches

Always glug and wipe

Remember LITTLE & OFTEN

Think mezze and tapas, not 5 courses

come up with an ALLERGY ALIBI

tell everyone you can't eat milk / bread / sausages then have your fill

STEP AWAY from the beetroot

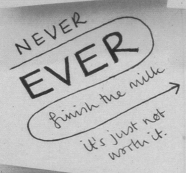

it's the foodie's anti-vandal paint

USE THE

So-and-so-came-round-and-all-they-could-eat-was-piccalilli-and-yoghurt

MANOEUVRE

RULER ☑
PROTRACTOR ☑
COMPASS ☑

put things back exactly where you found them

LIKE A CHEMISTRY LESSON, IT'S ALL ABOUT DILUTION...

→

(top things up with water)

PUT THE BALACLAVA DOWN

there's no need

# A Guide to Leaving notes →

**FED UP** with people "borrowing" your food & eating your special pie? Our Fridge Watch™ tips will stop your family/flatmates eating you out of house & home.

**CAPITAL LETTERS WERE MADE FOR THIS** LITTLE LETTERS JUST DON'T CUT THE MUSTARD (EVER DECREASING)

Don't write, 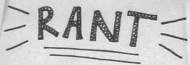 **RANT** And always use the passive aggressive

:( and !!!!! work a treat. As does underlining everything **TWICE!!!** :)

write a note in the **butter** with your finger. Simple and strangely satisfying.

name everything. **EVERYTHING**

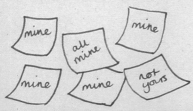
mine / mine / all mine / mine / mine / not yours

Replace ~~premium~~ with **value** (e.g. organic granola with no frills muesli. Just leave enough of the former to disguise the latter)

Set up a diversion  Leave your last rolo in the fridge

**TAKE THE BULB OUT OF THE FRIDGE & ALWAYS CARRY A TORCH**

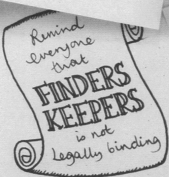
Remind everyone that **FINDERS KEEPERS** is not legally binding

"if all else fails" eat everything on the way home from the shop

# One cake wonder: big cake, small cakes, birthday cakes, fairy cakes

Cake is important. It makes birthdays edible, cups of tea ceremonial and everyone more friendly. So a dependable cake recipe is essential in life. This recipe makes one big cake or lots of little ones. There are loads of combinations, from simple to fancy. Just follow the basic mixes below and then embellish away.

Makes 1 big cake or
24 fairy cakes
250g unsalted butter, at room temperature
250g caster sugar (the unbleached golden stuff is best)
seeds from 1 vanilla pod
4 large free-range eggs
250g self-raising flour
2 tablespoons ground almonds

If you're making a big cake, you'll need two 23cm round loose-bottomed cake tins

If you're making small cakes, you'll need a muffin cake tin and 24 paper cases

Preheat your oven to 180°C/350°F/gas mark 4 and either grease your cake tin with butter or pop your paper cases into your cake tray.

Beat together the softened butter and the caster sugar till pale and fluffy. Then add the vanilla seeds and beat in the eggs, one at a time, adding a teaspoon of the flour with each egg.

Fold in the remaining flour, together with the ground almonds and mix well. Spoon the cake mix into the prepared tins or the paper cases (you'll need about 2 tablespoons per case) and bake in the oven. Try not to open the oven halfway through or your cakes may sink.

Big cakes: 25 to 30 minutes. Small cakes: about 15 to 20 minutes.

To test if your cakes are cooked, stick a metal skewer or the end of a teaspoon into them. If the cakes feel firm and the skewer/teaspoon comes out clean, they are ready to come out of the oven.

Once the cakes are out, be patient and allow them to cool completely on a wire rack. Otherwise your icing will be rubbish.

### Variations
- **Lemon:** Replace the vanilla with the zest of 2 lemons and the juice of 1 lemon.
- **Chocolate:** Replace the vanilla with 2 tablespoons of cocoa powder (or 3 if you want to go really chocolatey).
- **Coconut:** Replace the ground almonds with 2 tablespoons of desiccated coconut and the zest of 1 lime.

# AND TO TOP IT ALL OFF

A cake without a topping is like a dog wearing people clothes; not strictly wrong, but not quite right either. So here's a few of our favourite things to adorn the top of your cake with.

**Foolproof butter cream icing**  Cream 250g of butter, 1 teaspoon of vanilla essence and 200g of icing sugar until pale and fluffy. If you're going to make one of the alternative flavours below, add the extra bits at this point, minus the vanilla. Otherwise, add another 300g of icing sugar and beat well. If you're using an electric mixer or whisk, make sure it's on the slowest speed – you want to get as much air as possible into the icing to make it wispy and cloudlike.

**Chocolate**  Melt the butter with 100g of dark chocolate over a low heat. Then beat in the icing sugar as above.

**Strawberry**  Cream 150g of butter, then whizz up 150g strawberries, beat into the butter and mix in 500g of icing sugar as above.

**Chopped-up fresh fruit**  Raspberries, passion fruit, mango and strawberries are all perfect.

**Lemon**  Use 200g of butter and the zest of 2 lemons and then follow the method above.

**Crunchy nut**  Bashed up Crunchie bar or pistachio nuts work well sprinkled on top.

**Bountiful**  Scatter liberally with a handful of unsweetened desiccated coconut.

**Jam**  Spread on 4 big tablespoons of your favourite flavour.

**Whipped cream**  Gently whip 150ml of double cream into soft peaks and spread on top.

**Oranges or lemons**  Spread on 4 big tablespoons of your favourite curd.

**Berries**  Dot a handful of well placed whole strawberries or raspberries on top.

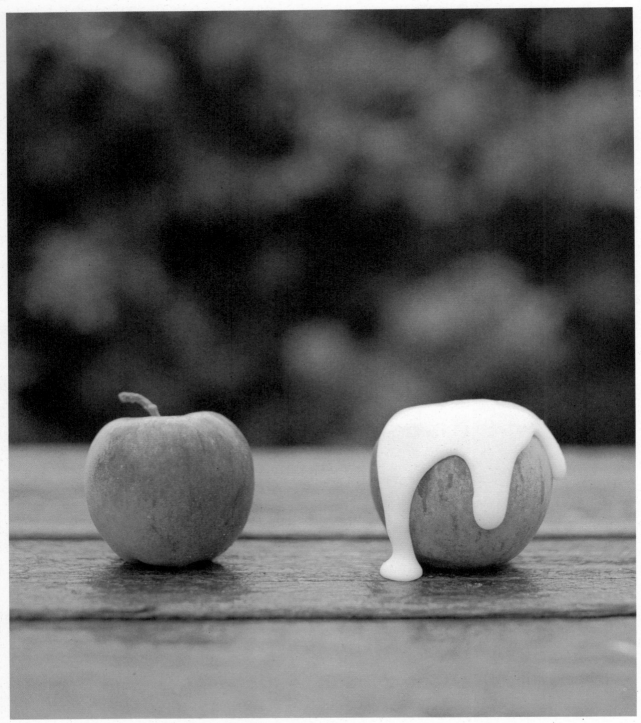

'I hate you, seagull.'

# Apple cake with honey icing

**A cake that takes no time to make, requires no special ingredients and slices up a treat for afternoon tea? Apple do nicely.**

Serves 8

For the cake
250g plain flour
½ teaspoon ground cinnamon
a pinch of grated nutmeg
1 ½ teaspoons baking powder
200ml olive oil
75g caster sugar
seeds from 1 vanilla pod
zest of 1 lemon
2 free-range eggs
2 apples, peeled, cored and
    chopped

For the honey icing
200g icing sugar
4 tablespoons lemon juice
4 tablespoons runny honey

Preheat your oven to 180°C/350°F/gas mark 4. You'll need two 23cm cake tins, buttered and the bases lined with greaseproof paper.

Mix the flour, cinnamon, nutmeg and baking powder in a bowl and set aside.

In a second bowl, whisk the oil, sugar, vanilla seeds and lemon zest. Now whisk in one of the eggs, followed by the apples, and mix again.

Start to add the flour bit by bit, whisking as you go, until you have a smooth batter. **Leave to stand.**

Separate the second egg and keep the yolk for another time (for example, for making mayonnaise). Put the egg white into a bowl and whisk until stiff peaks form. Carefully fold the whisked egg white into the batter. You want to be delicate here, to keep as much air in the mixture as possible.

Pour the mixture into the lined cake tins and bake for 30 to 35 minutes, until an inserted skewer comes out clean. Once golden on top, allow to cool on a rack while you make the icing.

Sieve the icing sugar into a mixing bowl and add the lemon juice bit by bit, followed by the honey. This is a loose icing that will dribble off the sides of your cake, so don't worry if it seems a little runny.

Once the cake is completely cool, dot a few holes across the top with a metal skewer and spoon the icing all over, allowing it to dribble down the sides and into the cake.

Keep for up to 5 days in an airtight container.

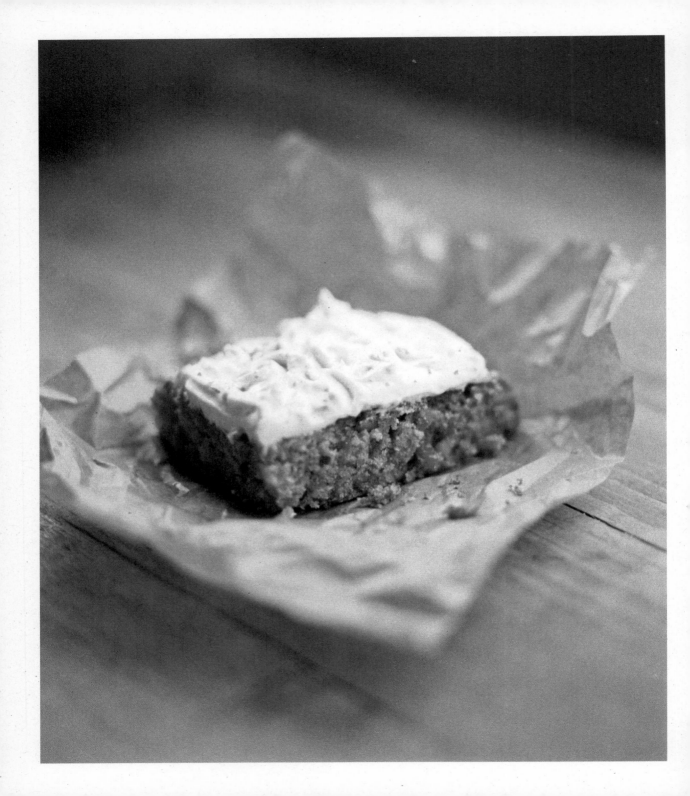

# Bronte's amazing carrot cake

Back in the early days of innocent, Bronte was the People team, the IT team, the Environment team, a bit of Finance and Head Cake Baker. In 2007, she left to open up the Scandinavian Kitchen (www.scandikitchen.co.uk), a cafe/shop in London where she sells good food from her homeland (Denmark) and its neighbours. If you're passing, pop in and try one of her cakes. If you're not, make this one.

Serves 16 (depending on how big you cut the slices)
counts towards your 5-a-day

**For the cake**
4 free-range eggs
200g soft brown sugar
200g golden caster sugar
1 teaspoon vanilla extract
400ml sunflower oil
400g self-raising flour
a pinch of salt
2 teaspoons ground cinnamon
1 teaspoon ground mixed spice
400g carrots, peeled and grated
150g pine nuts

**For the cream cheese icing**
300g cream cheese
zest and juice of 1 lime
100g icing sugar

**For the decoration (optional)**
grated carrot and toasted pine nuts

Preheat your oven to 180°C/350°F/gas mark 4 and line a cake tin with greaseproof paper (a rectangular 20 x 30cm tin is about right, or you can use a 25cm round tin).

Whisk the eggs, sugars, vanilla extract and sunflower oil together in a big mixing bowl.

Mix the flour, salt, cinnamon and mixed spice together in a second bowl and sift into the egg mixture. Fold the mixture together until the flour is well incorporated, then stir in the carrots and pine nuts.

Pour the cake mixture into the lined cake tin and bake in the middle of the oven for about 35 to 40 minutes, or until a skewer comes out clean.

While the cake is baking, make the icing. Whisk all ingredients together until fluffy. This icing is quite tart, so if you like yours a little sweeter, just add more icing sugar.

Allow the carrot cake to cool completely before spreading over the cream cheese icing and sprinkling with grated carrot and toasted pine nuts.

# Chocolate and beetroot brownies

Chocolate, vegetables and cake all happily co-existing in this dream of a brownie and gluten-free to boot? Pinch yourself. And then go and make a batch before the flying pigs start knocking.

**(Make sure you use cooked beetroots and not the pickled variety. Vinegar chocolate doesn't exist for a reason.)**

Makes about 24
counts towards your 5-a-day

200g unsalted butter
100g dark chocolate,
   broken up
200g golden caster sugar
2 tablespoons cocoa powder
3 free-range eggs
200g cooked and peeled
   beetroot, grated
100g ground almonds

Preheat your oven to 180°C/350°F/gas mark 4. Line a shallow baking tin with greaseproof paper.

Cut the butter into cubes, put it into a heatproof bowl with the chocolate and melt over a pan of simmering water, using a wooden spoon to prop the bowl above the water. Once melted, put to one side to cool a little.

In another bowl, mix together the sugar, cocoa powder and eggs and then stir this into the chocolate mix. Stir in the grated beetroot and ground almonds and fold the whole lot together. Don't mix it too much, though, or you'll end up with bouncy brownies, instead of the gooey variety.

Pour into the lined tray and bake for about 20 minutes, until just cooked – they should have a thin crust on top but still be a bit wobbly in the middle.

Leave in the tin for a few minutes before cutting into squares and transferring to a rack.

Serve the brownies warm, with a blob of crème fraîche and some grated orange zest, or crumble them over vanilla ice cream.

Store any leftovers in an airtight container for up to a week.

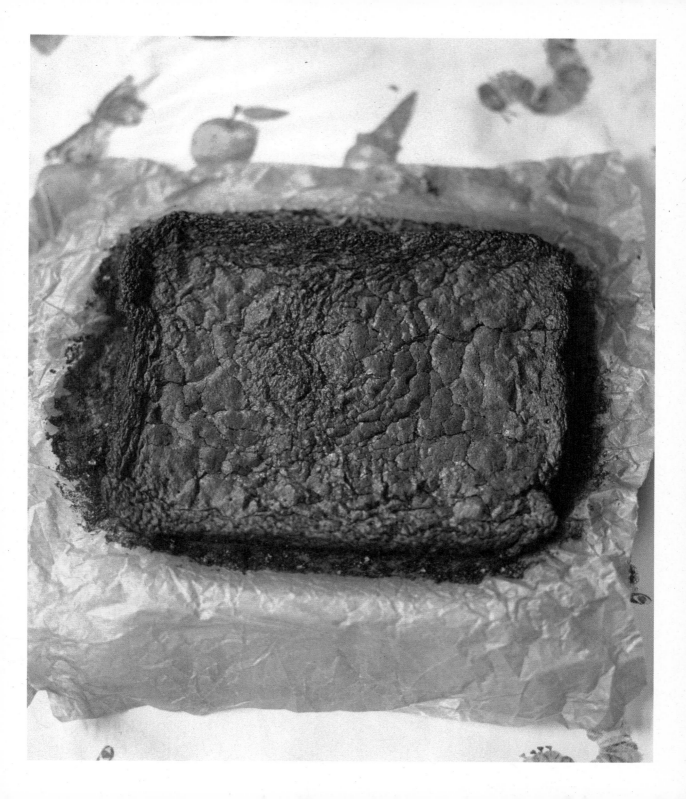

# Tiny banana and chocolate cookies

Egg-free, wheat-free, banana-full and chocolate-packed. It'll be a miracle if these cookies make it as far as tomorrow afternoon, let alone the cookie jar.

Makes about 25
counts towards your 5-a-day

3 ripe bananas, peeled
100g butter, melted and
   cooled
1 teaspoon vanilla extract, or
   the seeds from 1 vanilla pod
2 large handfuls of big fat
   porridge oats
100g ground almonds
100g unsweetened desiccated
   coconut
a handful of raisins or
   chopped dried apricots
a pinch of ground cinnamon
100g milk or plain chocolate,
   chopped into little bits

Preheat your oven to 180°C/350°F/gas mark 4. Line a baking sheet with greaseproof paper.

In a big mixing bowl, mash up the bananas with a fork. Add the melted butter and the vanilla and give it a good mix.

Put the rest of the ingredients except the chocolate into a bowl and stir in the banana mixture.

Now fold in the chocolate pieces. It won't look quite as firm as a normal cookie dough, but don't worry.

Space out the cookies (roughly 2 teaspoons per cookie) on the baking sheet so there's enough space for them to expand. Bake in the oven for about 30 minutes, until golden.

Leave them to cool for a few minutes on a wire rack, but not too long, as these are best eaten when the chocolate is still melty.

If there are any leftovers, store them in a tin for up to a week.

We say if. Good luck keeping these safe past teatime.

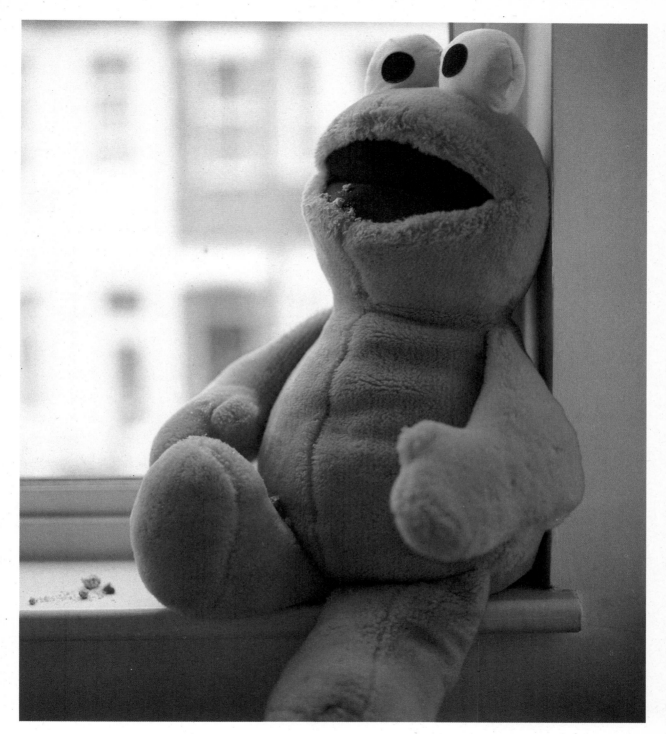

'Yes?'

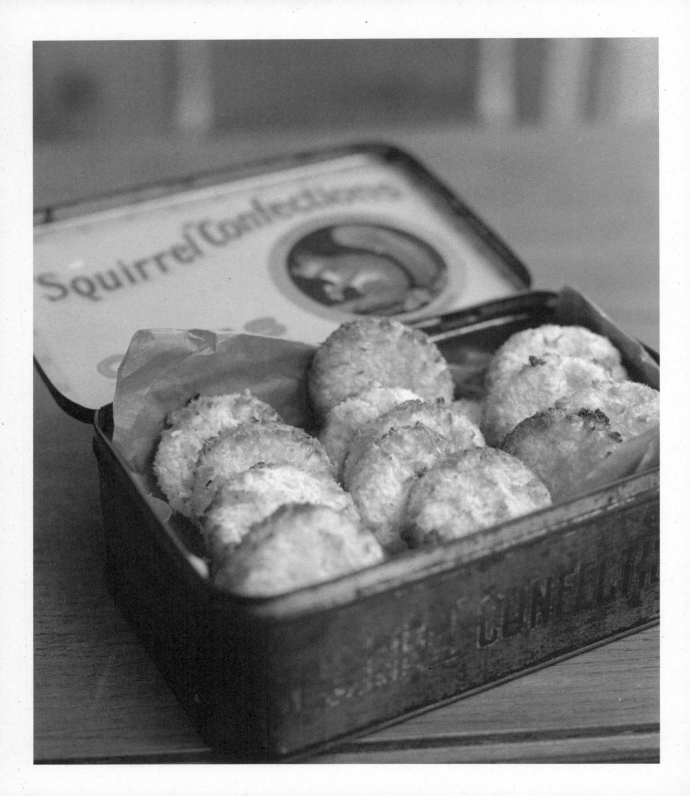

# Crumbs' coconut macaroons

Lucy and her sister, Claire, have a rather excellent blog (www.crumbsfood.co.uk) where they regularly jot down all the recipes they make for their kids. They've very kindly let us use their macaroon recipe in this book. These coconut bites of joy might look fiddly but they take mere minutes to make and even less time to eat. Gluten-free and seriously addictive. You've been warned.

Makes about 24
2 free-range eggs
100g caster sugar
160g desiccated coconut

Heat your oven to 180°C/350°F/gas mark 4. Lightly grease a baking tray.

Separate the eggs and put the yolks to one side for another day (you can use them to make mayonnaise, or add them to whole eggs for extra rich scrambled egg).

Mix the egg whites, sugar and coconut in a bowl with a spoon until well-combined and then pour the mixture on to a clean worktop.

Shape into a rectangle and press down with your hands to flatten to about 1cm thick.

Use a small biscuit cutter or glass (about 4cm in diameter) to cut out rounds and place them on the baking tray.

Bake in the oven for 12 to 15 minutes, until golden. Cool on a wire rack and store in an airtight container for up to a week.

# Chocolate bran flake cakes

This is Ceri's mum Sian's healthier, crunchier version of the classic jumble sale chocolate cornflake cake. They take about 6 minutes to make, have a wonderfully malty taste and are great for rainy day treats, birthday parties and all good church hall bring-and-buys.

Makes about 12
100g butter
4 tablespoons runny honey or golden syrup
6 tablespoons cocoa powder
150g bran flakes

Melt the butter, honey/syrup and cocoa powder in a big pan over a very low heat until the butter has melted and the mixture is smooth. You're aiming for a sauce that isn't too runny, so add more honey/syrup or cocoa powder if needed.

Stir in the bran flakes without bashing them up and spoon the mixture into paper cases or on to a lightly buttered tray.

Pop them into the fridge for 20 to 30 minutes to set. Once they're firm to touch, they're good to goo (sorry).

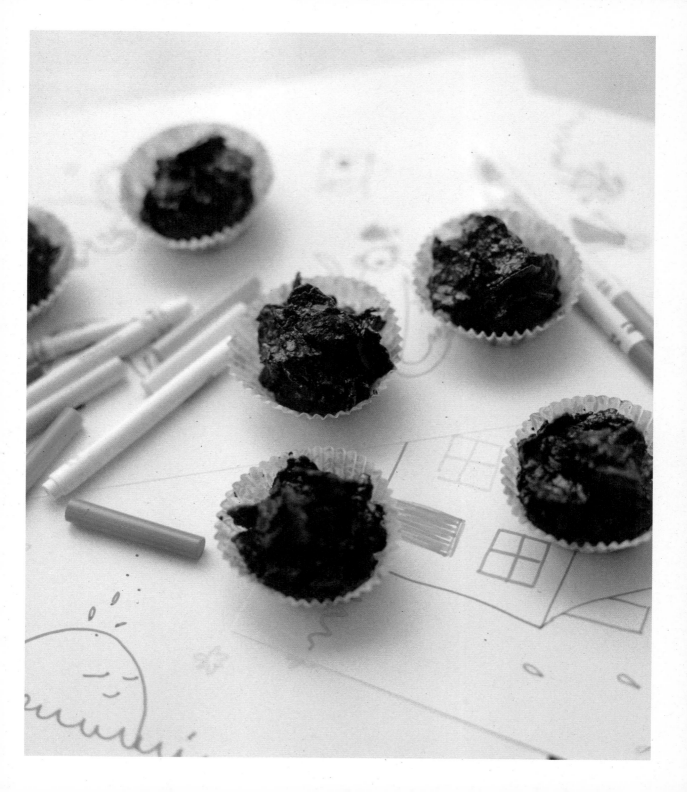

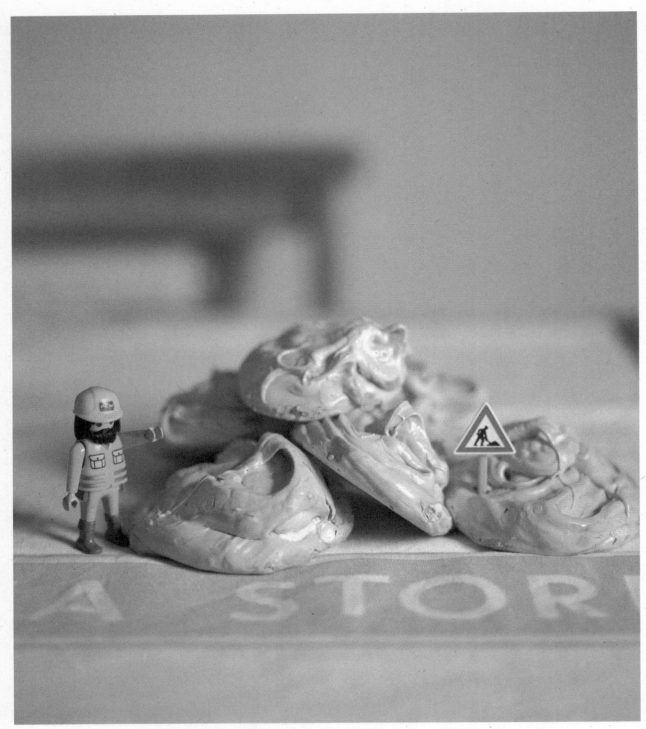

'Tim, stop making such a pavlova of everything and hand me that spade.'

# Brown sugar meringues

This recipe uses brown sugar as it makes for more caramelly, gooey meringues. They'll keep in a container for a couple of weeks and are a simple way to jazz up after-dinner fruit.

Preheat your oven to 150°C/300°F/gas mark 2.

Separate the eggs and put the yolks to one side. (You can use them for mayonnaise, custard or to yellow up an omelette.)

In a clean bowl, whisk the egg whites until they form firm peaks, like little snowy mountains.

Add the sugar and a pinch of salt and whisk on the highest setting your mixer or arm has for about 5 minutes, until all the grains of sugar have disappeared.

Line a baking tray with greaseproof paper and spoon on the mixture in blobs (about 2 good tablespoonfuls per blob).

Bake in the oven for 45 minutes, until golden and crunchy on the outside, chewy on the inside.

Stuff to serve your meringues with
- Try using them for fruit mess (page 256) or crumbled up in quick banana ice cream (page 254)

- For a slightly more wintry affair, whip up some double cream with 1 teaspoon of icing sugar and a pinch of ground cinnamon and serve with the meringues and tinned or poached pears. Or try the fruit compote in the easy rice pudding recipe (page 259).

- Make one big meringue. It'll take about an hour to cook. Then fill it with fruit and crème fraîche and you've got a pavlova.

Serves 8
4 free-range eggs
200g soft brown or light
   muscovado sugar
a pinch of salt

# THINGS TO DO IN (60) Minutes

While you're waiting for the roast to roast

## WRITE A LETTER

### USING CUTOUTS FROM THE NEWSPAPER

NAME YOUR FUTURE KIDS. IF YOU ALREADY HAVE KIDS, NAME YOUR FUTURE PETS.

WASH THE CAR

RECORD YOUR OWN RADIO SHOW AND INVITE SPECIAL GUESTS

MAKE A BIRD HOUSE

CHEEP

OH WOW

HAVE A NAP

MAKE PASTA JEWELLERY

Draw a comic

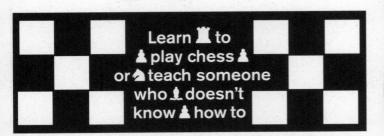

Learn ♜ to ♟ play chess ♟ or ♟ teach someone who ♟ doesn't know ♟ how to

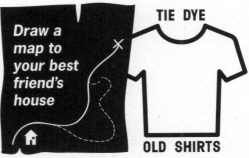

Draw a map to your best friend's house

TIE DYE

OLD SHIRTS

PAINT ONE WALL IN YOUR ROOM

Write until your pen has run out
Write until your pen has run out
Write until your pen has run out
Write until your pen has run out...

Get properly stuck into a book

① WRITE A LIST OF 10 THINGS THAT YOU'VE ALWAYS WANTED TO KNOW...

② ...THEN GO AND FIND OUT ALL THE ANSWERS BY ANY MEANS NECESSARY

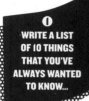

Go through and organise all the photos on your camera memory card

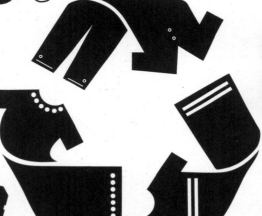

SORT OUT OLD CLOTHES FOR RECYCLING

Write a short story. If you can't think of anything to write about, go to the park and write about people you see.

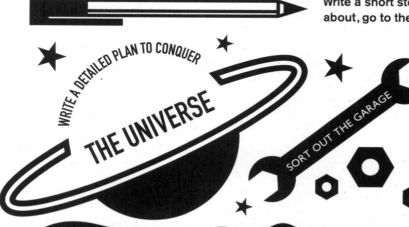
WRITE A DETAILED PLAN TO CONQUER THE UNIVERSE

SORT OUT THE GARAGE

MAKE A → TREASURE HUNT FOR YOUNGER SIBLINGS →

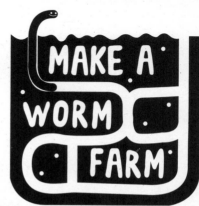
MAKE A WORM FARM

# Traffic-light ketchup

Red, yellow, green, orange, red, yellow, orange, yellow, red, green, yellow – all depends on what colour tomatoes you end up using.

If you're using different coloured tomatoes, make sure to divide the sauce into 3 and then you can make 3 different colours at once.

Makes 2 big bottles
counts towards your 5-a-day

1 red onion, peeled
1 carrot, peeled
1 stick of celery, peeled
a small piece of fresh ginger,
   peeled and grated
2 garlic cloves, peeled and
   grated
2 cloves
½ a cinnamon stick
1 teaspoon smoked paprika
1 teaspoon coriander seeds
olive oil
1kg ripe tomatoes (red, yellow
   or green)
a few sprigs of basil, leaves
   picked
200ml red wine vinegar
150g brown sugar

Use a grater or food processor to grate all the veg, along with the ginger and garlic.

Put the grated veg, ginger, garlic and spices into a big pan with a splash of olive oil and cook on a low heat for about 10 minutes. While the veg are cooking, roughly chop the tomatoes.

*If you're using different coloured tomatoes, remember to divide the sauce here.*

Once the veg in the pan is soft, add the tomatoes along with a mug of water and allow to simmer for another 10 minutes, until the sauce has thickened.

Stir in the basil and take off the heat. Either blitz the sauce up in a food processor or use a potato masher to give it a really good bash.

Once bashed, push the whole lot through a sieve using a wooden or metal spoon.

Once sieved, return the sauce to the pan, add the vinegar and sugar and simmer until it has a ketchup consistency.

Store in the fridge for a couple of weeks, or pour into sterilised bottles, seal tightly and keep in the fridge for up to 2 months.

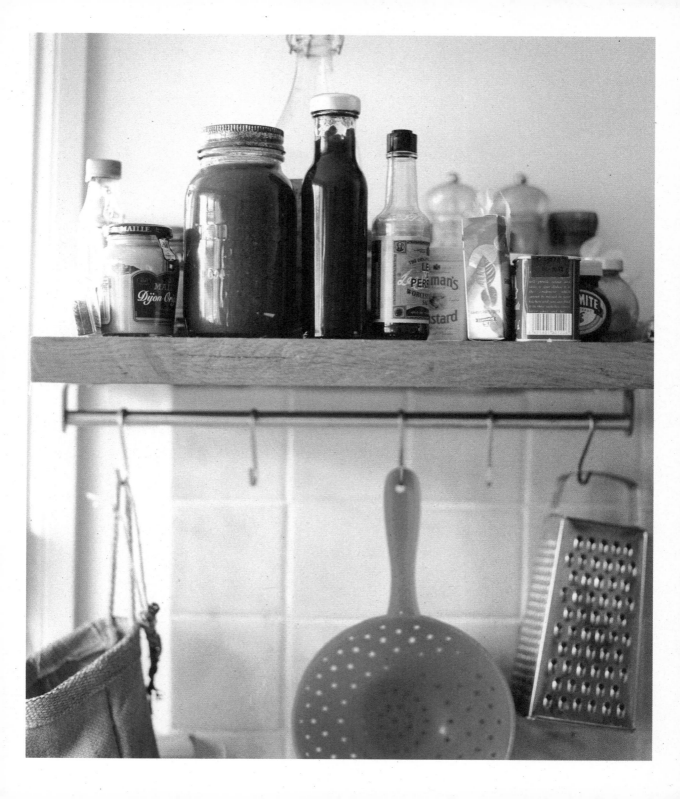

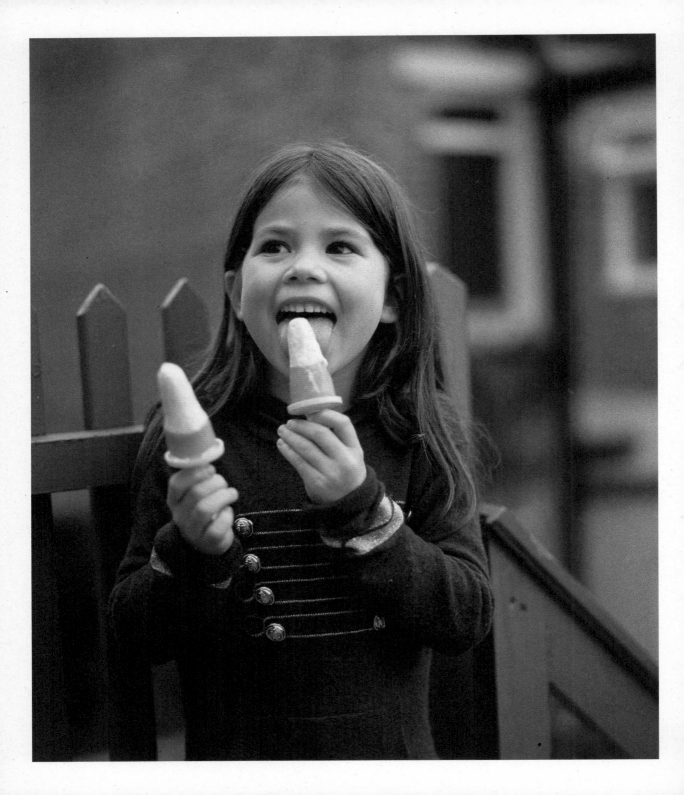

# Rhubarb and custard ice lollies

Despite its pudding history, rhubarb is actually a vegetable, distantly related to sorrel and the sea grape (whatever that is). Rhubarb is a fine provider of vitamin C and packed full of fibre. It's also bright pink – making sneaking all that good stuff into these lollies far easier than trying to pass off salty grape ice cream as tasty. When it comes to custard, you can use homemade or ready-made. They both work a treat.

Makes 8 lollies
counts towards your 5-a-day

8 lolly moulds (or glasses and lolly sticks)
500g homemade or ready-made vanilla custard
4 sticks of rhubarb, trimmed
2 tablespoons caster sugar
juice of 1 orange

Depending on the size of your lolly moulds or glasses, half fill each one with custard and put them into the freezer while you cook the rhubarb.

Cut the rhubarb into 2.5cm pieces and put into a pan with the sugar, orange juice and a splash of water. Simmer over a low heat until you have a thick pink purée. Allow to cool, then fill up the moulds with the rhubarb. If you've got more time, you can make your lollies stripy by layering up the two mixtures bit by bit. Or you can use pure rhubarb, or pure custard. Depending on your lolly taste.

# Simple custard

Still one of the best things to pour over your puddings and a genius way of using up egg yolks.

Serves 4–6
250ml milk
250ml single cream
seeds of 1 vanilla pod
2 tablespoons of golden caster sugar
6 large free-range egg yolks

Put the milk, cream, vanilla seeds, vanilla pod and half the sugar into a saucepan over a low heat. Bring to the boil, then take off the heat and allow to cool. Whisk the egg yolks in a bowl with the rest of the sugar until pale and creamy. Remove the vanilla pod from the milk then gradually add the milk to the yolk bowl, whisking as you go. Then pour it all back into the saucepan over a low heat, stirring with a wooden spoon for 5–10 minutes as your custard thickens. Don't be tempted to turn up the heat. Just keep stirring and if you get any lumpy bits, sieve them out at the end.

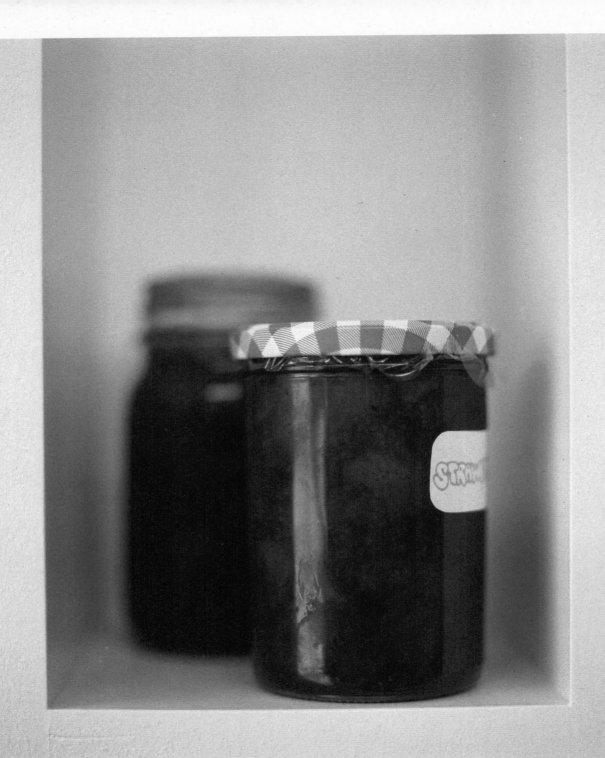

# Super-quick strawberry jam

You can easily use this method for other fruits – raspberries, plums, gooseberries, rhubarb. You'll just need to add a bit more sugar as these fruits tend to be slightly more tart. Which, along with toast and crumpets, is another good thing to spread your jam on.

Makes about 6 jars
1kg bright red ripe strawberries, washed and stalks removed
500g golden refined caster sugar
seeds from 1 vanilla pod
juice of 1 big lemon

First you need to sterilise your jars. Wash them thoroughly, then either put them into the oven at 110°C/225°F/gas mark ¼ for 20 minutes, or immerse them in boiling water for 10 minutes. Alternatively you can run them through a hot programme in the dishwasher.

Put the strawberries into a bowl with the sugar, vanilla seeds and lemon juice and use a potato masher to give them a good mashing.

Put the whole lot into a big pan and bring to the boil. Once boiling, turn down the heat and simmer for about 5 minutes, then remove from the heat. Use a ladle to skim off the pink foamy stuff and leave to cool.

Once the jam has cooled, check its consistency by putting a spoonful on a cold plate. It should be not too runny and not too thick. If it's very runny, heat it up again and then leave to cool.

When you're happy with your jam, spoon it into the jars and top with a little circle of jam paper. Seal tightly, write the date and jam name on a label and store in a cool dark place until toast time.

# GOOD THINGS TO

---

# DRINK

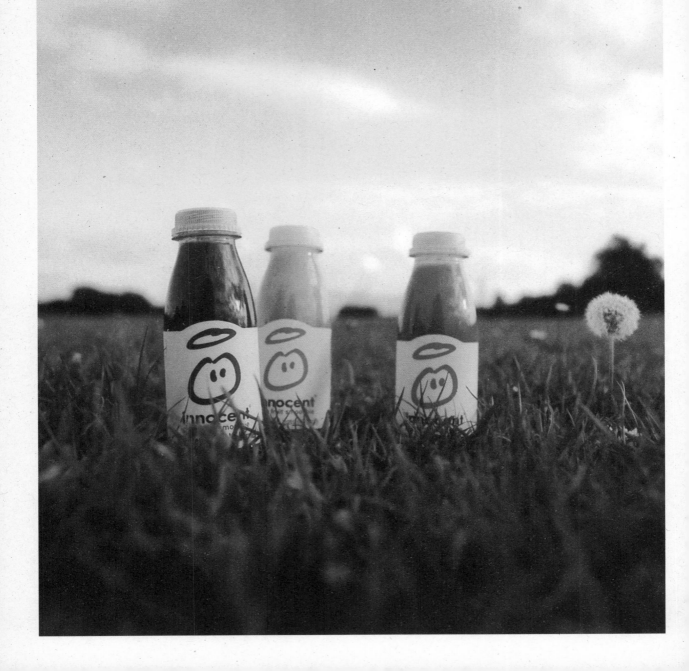

We've been making drinks for a long time. Some of these recipes you might have tried. Others you might not. We've mixed up old with new, simple with fancy. So please go forth and blend.

# Classic all-rounders

Crowd pleasers every time.

## Strawberry and banana

Serves 1 generously
2 portions of your 5-a-day

2½ apples
½ an orange
7 strawberries
juice of ½ a banana, peeled

An old one but a family favourite, a timeless combination and the exact same recipe you'll find in our bottles. Please enjoy repeatedly.

Cut the apples into wedges and put them through a juicer. Squeeze the juice from the orange half. Pour the apple juice and orange juice into a blender. Add the strawberries and banana and whizz away.

## Blackberry and blueberry

Serves 1 generously
2 portions of your 5-a-day

2½ apples
1 punnet of blueberries
1 punnet of blackberries
½ a banana, peeled
½ an orange

To be enjoyed on the days when the sun is shining, the birds are singing and the hedgerows are bursting with blackberries/handily packaged punnets of blueberries.

Cut the apples into wedges and put them through a juicer. Pour the juice into a blender. Add the berries and banana with a dash of freshly squeezed OJ and whizz until you get the desired consistency.

## Orange, banana and pineapple

Serves 2 generously
2 portions of your 5-a-day

1 succulent pineapple
1 orange, juiced
1 banana, peeled
a wedge of lime

This was one of the first recipes we ever made and, like a trusty dog, it stuck with us through good times, bad times and dodgy haircuts. You can no longer get it in our little bottles, so we thought we'd bring it back from pasture to be enjoyed again. Unlike the permed mullet undercut of 2005. Only the barber found that one amusing.

Peel and core the pineapple. Put half the pineapple through a juicer. Cut the other half into chunks and put them into a blender. Add the orange juice to the blender with the pineapple juice and the banana. Add a squeeze of lime juice and whizz until smooth.

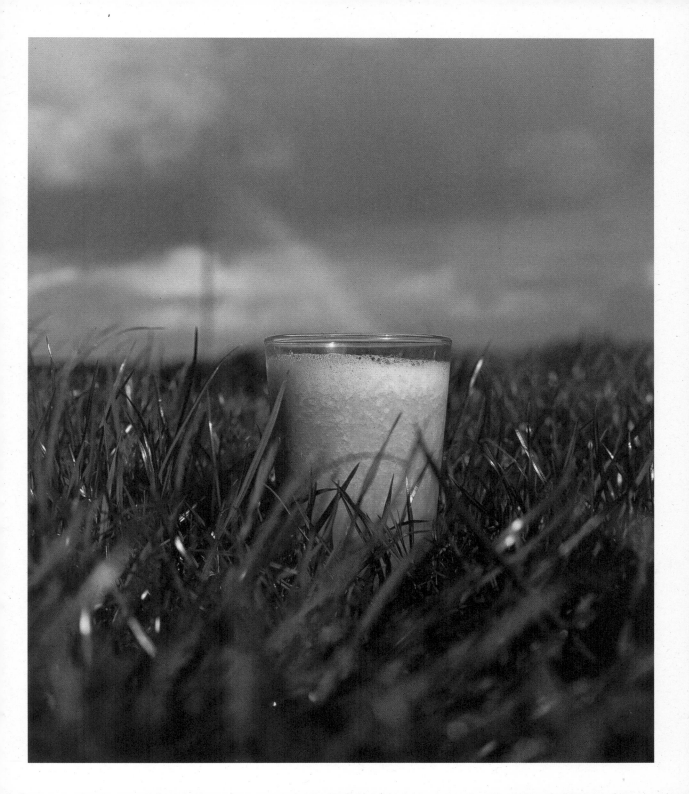

# Whingy?

Here are some ways to silence the 'I'm hungry' chorus.

## Banana and cinnamon thickie

Everything a good thickie should be. Creamy, tasty and a bit speckly.

Cut the apple into wedges and put them through a juicer. Pour the juice into a blender and add the other ingredients. Whizz until smooth.

Sneak 50ml bottled, freshly pressed apple juice into the drink if you can't be bothered to press the apple yourself.

Serves 1
2 portions of your 5-a-day

1 apple (Royal Gala if possible)
2 bananas, peeled
4 tablespoons plain yoghurt
1 teaspoon honey
½ teaspoon freshly ground cinnamon

## Peanut butter and banana lumpie

Lumpie rather than smoothie as it's a bit more, well, lumpy. Great as a mid-morning snack to see you through to lunchtime.

Put everything in a blender and whizz. Drink. Repeat as required.

Serves 1
1 portion of your 5-a-day

1 medium banana, peeled
3 tablespoons plain yoghurt
125ml milk
1 tablespoon crunchy peanut butter

## White chocolate smoothie

Very thick and very rich, this recipe could be likened to drinking a white fluffy cloud. Or describing certain pop stars.

Melt the chocolate in a heatproof bowl set over a pan of simmering water. Pour the melted chocolate into a blender and add the honey, grapes and banana. Cut the apple into wedges and put them into a juicer, then add the juice to the blender and whizz it up. Cool in the fridge before drinking and serve in an ice-cold glass. It's important to chill the glass or the melted chocolate makes it too warm.

(This recipe was kindly sent to us by Nadine Akle, innocent drinker and recipe thinker. Thank you very, very much.)

Serves 1
2 portions of your 5-a-day

6 (yes, 6 is enough) chunks of white chocolate
1 teaspoon runny honey
a small bunch of white grapes
1 banana, peeled
1 sharp apple (Granny Smith or Cox's would be nice)

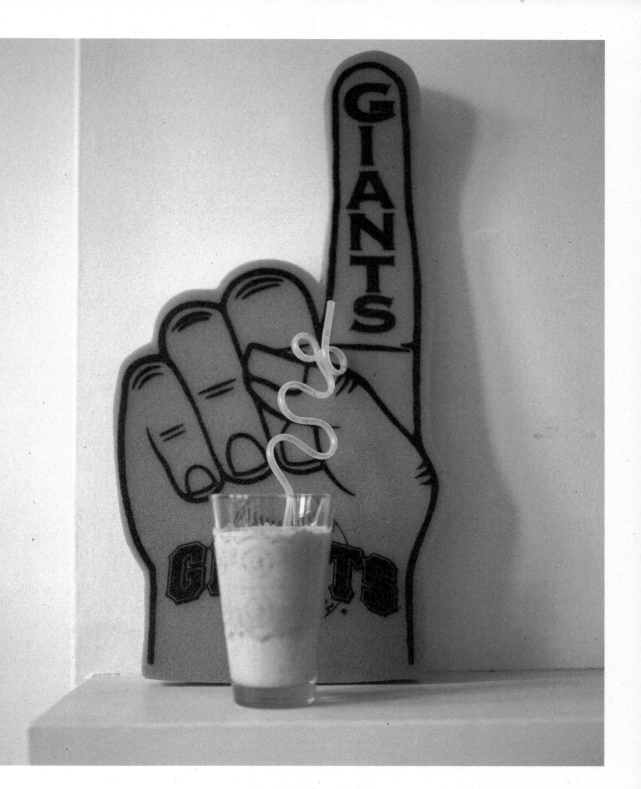

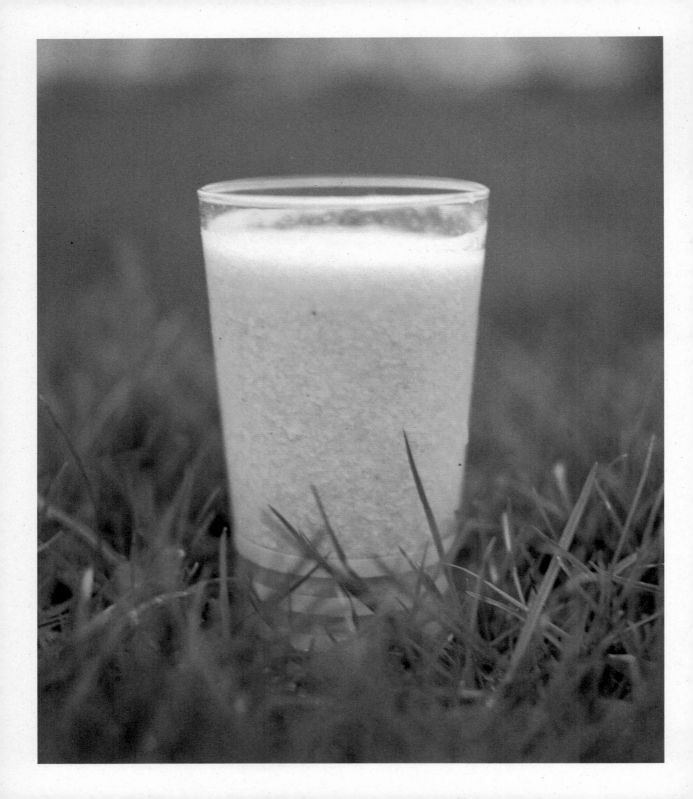

# Poorly?

TLC in a glass.

## Apple, banana, pineapple and lemon

Serves 1 generously
2 portions of your 5-a-day

1 apple (preferably Russet)
1 lemon
1 banana, peeled
¼ of a pineapple
1 person to make this drink
  for you

Tastier than that pink aniseedy stuff, this nutrient-rich recipe is great for settling dicky tums. And seeing as you should be able to find these ingredients all year round, there are no excuses for resorting to pink gloop.

Cut the apple into wedges and put them through a juicer. Pour the juice into a blender. Squeeze the lemon and pour the juice into the blender, adding the banana too. Remove the skin from the pineapple and slice the flesh. Add to the blender and whizz everything until smooth. Serve over ice, or add 4 or 5 ice cubes to the blender.

50ml bottled, freshly pressed apple juice will do if your juicer is on strike.

## Hot lemon, honey and ginger – served warm

Serves 2
1 unwaxed lemon
2.5cm of fresh ginger
6 teaspoons Manuka honey

As tasty as it is toasty, this is the hot toddy of the smoothie world. The original recipe uses Manuka honey because of its anti-bacterial properties, but the regular stuff will do just as well. It also tastes just as good chilled. In case you were wondering.

Squeeze half the lemon and pour the juice into a mug. Slice the other half of the lemon. Peel and finely slice the ginger. Add the ginger, lemon slices and honey to the mug. Pour on the boiling water, leave to infuse and cool for 5 minutes.

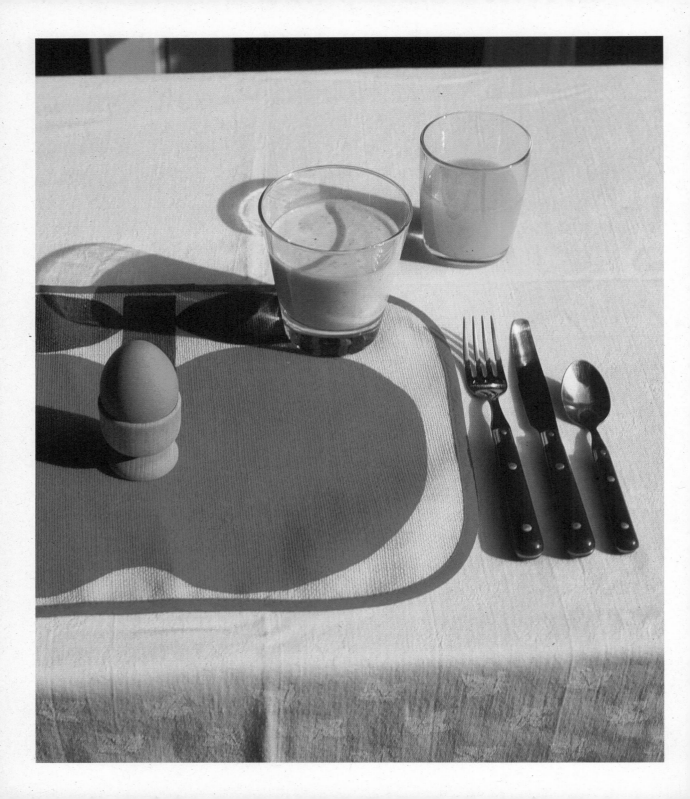

# Slept in?

Liquid breakfast. Down in one. Or three.

## Strawberry and banana lumpie

Serves 1 generously or
2 as a snack
2 portions of your 5-a-day

5 strawberries
1 medium banana, peeled
4 tablespoons plain yoghurt
a couple of splashes of milk
1 teaspoon clear honey
1 tablespoon rolled oats
1 tablespoon wheat flakes
1 tablespoon raisins

**The original breakfast in a cup – fruit, yoghurt and fibre. You'll be full, very happy and you might even be able to squeeze past 11 a.m. without wanting to eat your sandwiches.**

Destalk the strawberries. Place the banana, strawberries, yoghurt, milk and honey into a blender and whizz until smooth. Add the oats, wheat flakes and raisins (or substitute muesli for these three) and whizz to the desired consistency.

Watch out for muesli with added sugar. You shouldn't really need it – the honey and raisins are naturally sweet enough.

## Banana, oats and medjool dates

Serves 2
1½ portions of your 5-a-day

2 apples
½ a banana, peeled
2 teaspoons acacia honey
3 medjool dates
200g yoghurt
20g oats

**No time for porridge? Get your oats-to-go. With bananas, honey and sweet, malty dates, you might say that this is the best breakfast drink on earth. Or at least a very tasty way to start the day.**

Cut the apples into wedges and put them through a juicer. Pour the juice into a blender, add the banana, honey and dates and whizz until smooth. Add the yoghurt and oats and pulse 4 times.

# the innocent wee-ometer™

Smoothies and juices are great, but we all know you're supposed to drink a bit of water too. An easy way to check that you're getting enough water is to use our patented innocent wee-ometer™. Just compare your wee to what's on the chart – the darker your wee, the more water you need to drink. A nice pale yellow (Wee Nirvana®) is what you should be aiming for.

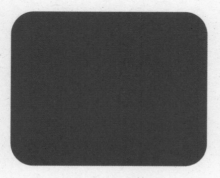

A night out with
Keith Richards

Office party

No one can see the smell
of asparagus

Half a shandy

'Blow into the bag
please, Sir'

Beetroot surprise

Wee Nirvana®

I can pee clearly now

# Sleepy?

Perfect just before bed or for the nights when the sheep just keep coming.

## Boozy milk

Serves 2
250ml milk
2 capfuls of dark rum
1 teaspoon runny honey
freshly ground cinnamon,
   to taste
1 settee

Embrace winter and the long, dark nights it brings by heating up a nice, warming mug of boozy milk before you go to bed. Better still, pop your pyjamas on the minute you get home and make a proper night of it. For grown-ups only.

Put the milk, rum and honey into a saucepan and whisk over a low heat until warm. Pour into your favourite mug. Sprinkle with cinnamon.

Feeling lazy? Don't want a dirty pan? Then pour all the ingredients into a microwave-friendly jug, whisk and microwave for 1 to 1½ minutes. For ground cinnamon, get some cinnamon sticks and grind them into dust using a pestle and mortar. Or cheat and consult your spice rack.

## Non-boozy milk

Serves 2
250ml milk
2 cardamom pods
2 cloves
1 teaspoon brown sugar
freshly ground cinnamon, to
   taste

Almost as relaxing as boozy milk, but for drivers and all those under 18.

Put all the ingredients except the cinnamon into a saucepan and whisk lightly over a low heat until warm. Remove the cardamom pods and cloves, unless you like chewing on them. Pour into your second-favourite mug. Sprinkle with cinnamon.

Want to make the drink during the ad break? Then pour all the ingredients into a microwave-proof jug, whisk and microwave for 1 to 1½ minutes.

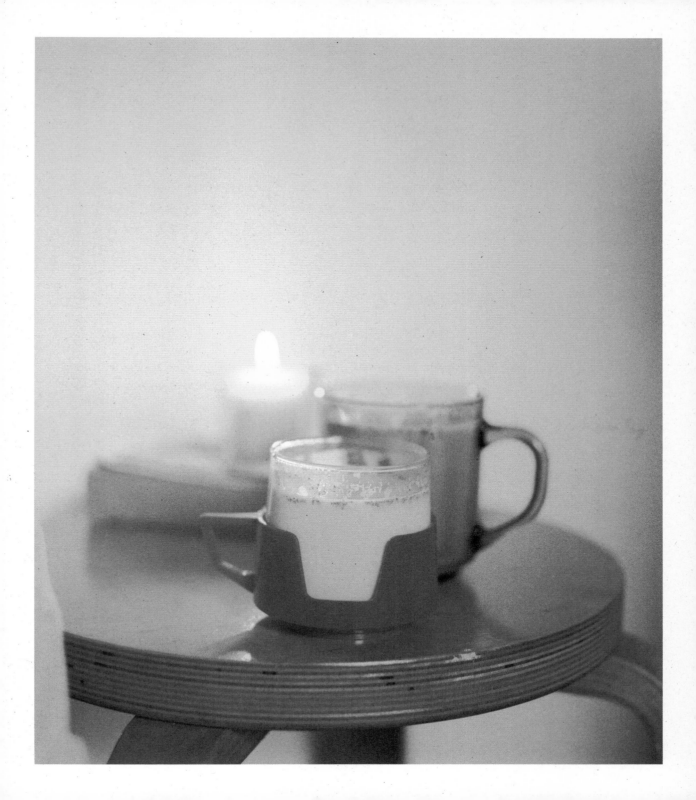

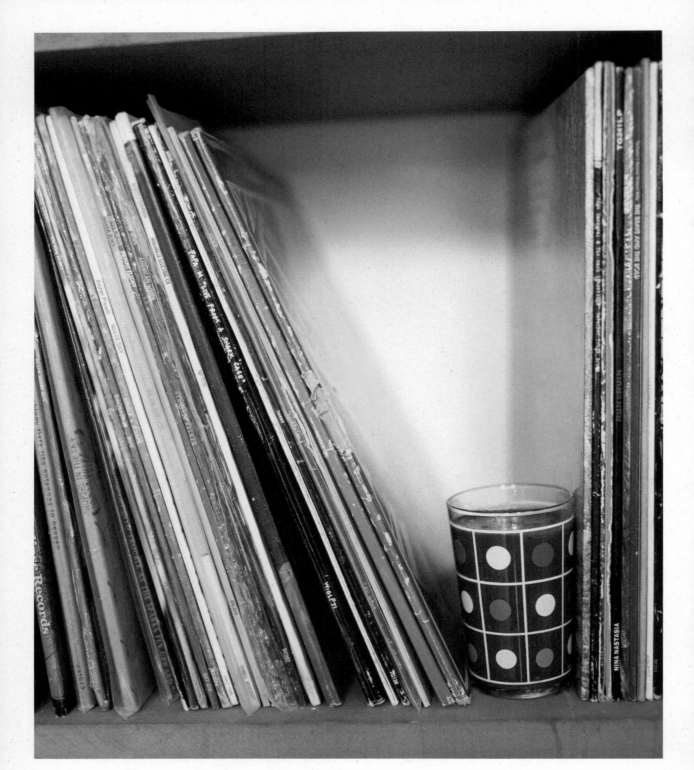

## Blackberry and lavender

Serves 2
1 portion of your 5-a-day

2 apples
8 plump blackberries
3 teaspoons lavender honey
200g plain yoghurt

Calming lavenderzzzzz...

Cut the apples into wedges, put them through a juicer and pour the juice into the blender. Add the blackberries and honey to the blender and blend until mixed. Add the yoghurt and pulse twice.

## Dark chocolate and cherry

Serves 2
1½ portions of your 5-a-day

2 apples
10 cherries
½ a banana, peeled
50g dark chocolate

**Total liquid decadence that tastes even better when someone else makes it for you. Simply leave the page open with all the ingredients next to it, recline gracefully on the chaise longue and refuse to do anything till it's handed to you in a goblet with a straw.**

Cut the apples into wedges, put them through a juicer and pour the juice into a blender. Chop up the cherries, discarding the stones. Slice the banana and add it to the blender with the cherries. Whizz everything together. Melt the chocolate over a pan of simmering water, then add the melted chocolate to the rest of the blended ingredients and give it all a final whizz.

# Sneaky?

Smuggle in more good stuff with these hide-and-seek made drinkable recipes.

## Rhubarb and custard

Serves 2
2 portions of your 5-a-day

2 large apples (Russet would be best)
3 large sticks of rhubarb
4 tablespoons custard
1 small piece of chopped stem ginger

Fibre-packed rhubarb, juicy apples and a dose of vitamin C, all mixed together with creamy custard for what is known in all our houses as pudding-in-a-glass.

Cut the apples into wedges and put them through a juicer. Cut the rhubarb into chunks and place in a saucepan with the apple juice. Cover and stew over a gentle heat for 5 or 6 minutes, until the rhubarb is soft. Leave it to cool. When the rhubarb and apple are cool, pour them into a blender. Add the custard and ginger and blend until smooth.

You can use any kind of custard to make this recipe. We made our own from scratch (page 313), but the ready-made or powdered variety made with milk work just as well.

## Black apples

Serves 2
2 portions of your 5-a-day

2 apples
50 blackcurrants
2 apricots
1 teaspoon black treacle

This recipe was kindly given to us by Lizzie Vann, the founder of Baby Organix, and featured in our last smoothie recipe book. Lizzie assures us it's the perfect drink to make sure the small people in your life grow up big and strong. Drink up.

Cut the apples into wedges and put them through a juicer. Put the apple juice, blackcurrants, stoned apricots and treacle into a blender and whizz until smooth.

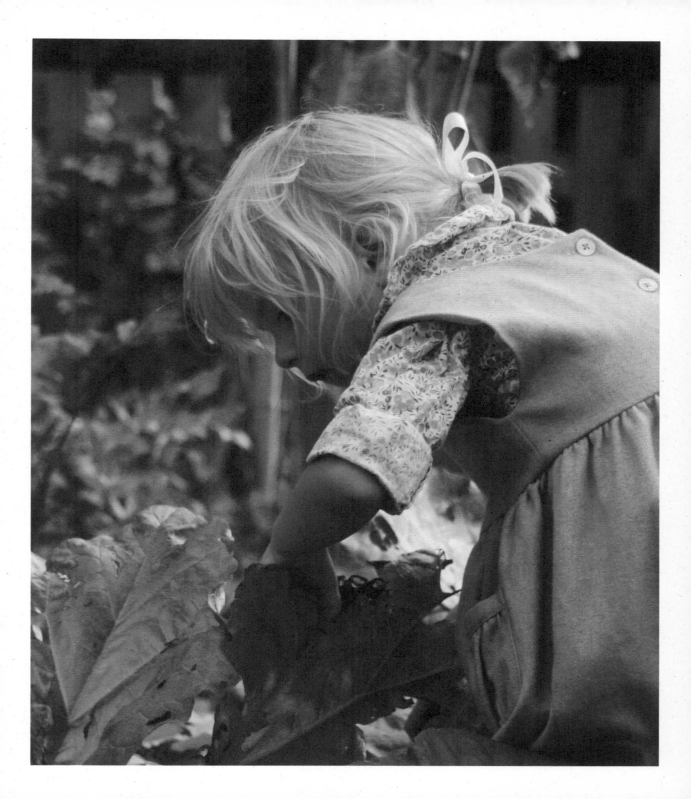

## Mango, passion fruit and squash

Serves 1
2 portions of your 5-a-day

½ a juicy mango
½ a banana, peeled
2½ apples
½ a passion fruit
½ an orange
2 tablespoons cooked mashed
   butternut squash/sweet
   potato/pumpkin

Squash? What squash? Thanks to Mother Nature being savvy on her colour scheme, smuggling in leftovers has never been so easy (or tasty).

Peel the mango and slice it into the blender. Pop the banana into the blender as well. Cut the apples into wedges and put them through the juicer. Strain the juice from the passion fruit (don't add the seeds) into the blender, using a sieve. Add the apple juice and the juice of half an orange to the blender. Then add the squash and whizz everything until smooth. Pour over ice and sip.

## Beetroot, pear and apple fizz

Serves 2
2 portions of your 5-a-day

1 small raw beetroot
1 apple
1 pear
a squeeze of lemon
fizzy water

Looks like purple lemonade, tastes like pear and apple juice and turns your wee pink. Magic stuff indeed.

Top and tail the beetroot, peel and cut into chunks, then slice the apple and pear into wedges. Put everything through a juicer, stir in the lemon juice and then top up with fizzy water.

## Melon and berries

Serves 2
2 portions of your 5-a-day

1 apple
½ a Galia melon
1 wedge of watermelon
½ a pink grapefruit
½ a banana, peeled
2 handfuls of frozen mixed
   berries

When you tire of tumblers or normal glasses, you can drink this out of a melon cup. Just scoop out the seeds of the other half of your Galia melon, pour your smoothie into the well and add two straws. Glassware c/o M Nature.

Cut the apple into wedges and put them through a juicer. Remove the seeds and skin from the melons, slice the flesh into wedges and put them through the juicer. Squeeze the grapefruit. Put the melon, apple and grapefruit juice into a blender with the banana and the berries and whizz until smooth.

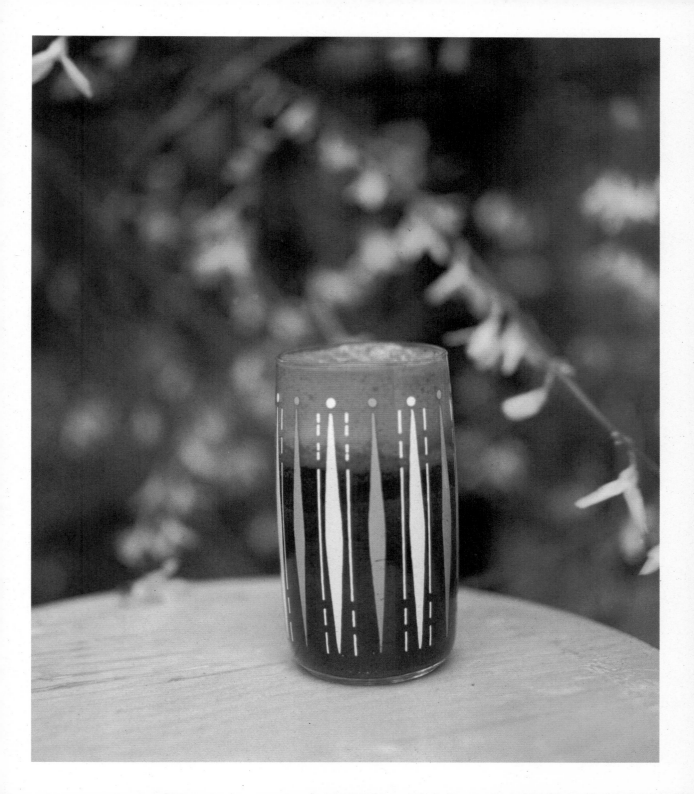

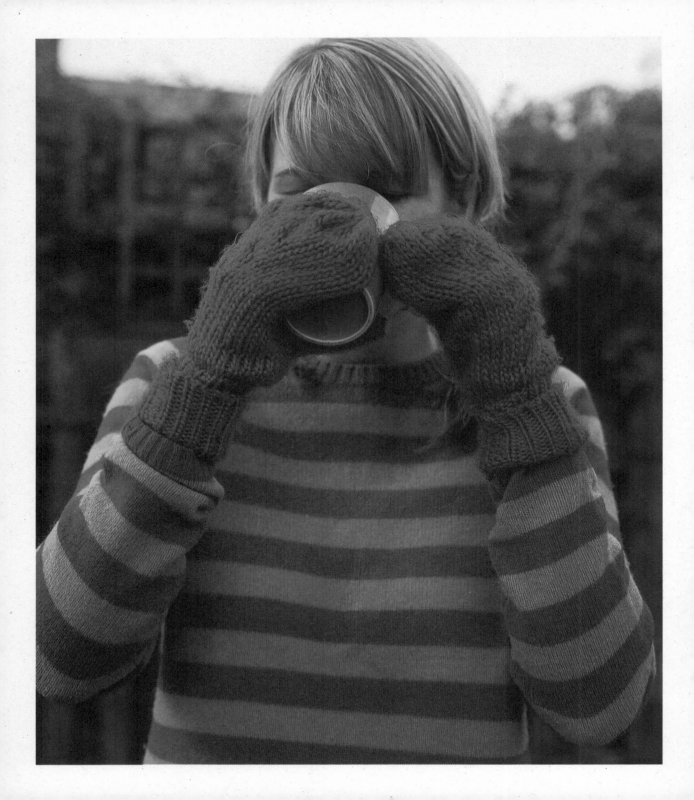

# Nippy out?

Warm your cockles with these or try a mug of lemon, honey and ginger (page 325).

## Hot apple and cinnamon

Serves 1

1 portion of your 5-a-day

3 apples or cloudy apple juice
1 teaspoon ground cinnamon

**This is another recipe from the good ladies at Crumbs (www.crumbsfood.co.uk). Great for frosty mornings.**

If you're making your own apple juice, cut the apples into wedges and put them through a juicer. Then pour the juice into a small pan, stir in the cinnamon and gently heat. Pour into a mug.

Feeling fancy? Pop in a cinnamon stick while warming the apple juice to let it infuse. Or add a squeeze of lemon juice and a drizzle of honey or maple syrup for a sweeter treat.

## Bonfire juice (a.k.a. apple juice for adults)

Makes 8 big glasses

1 portion of your 5-a-day (if made with apple juice)

1½ litres dry cider or cloudy apple juice
zest of 1 orange, pared into strips
4 cinnamon sticks
4 cloves
¼ teaspoon grated nutmeg
2 tablespoons brown sugar
a splash of rum or apple brandy (or maple syrup for non-boozy)

**Warm spicy cider. Yum. Replace the booze with cloudy apple juice for kids and drivers.**

Pour the cider or apple juice into a large saucepan and add everything else, apart from the rum. Heat gently for 20 minutes but don't boil. Add the rum or maple syrup, strain if you like and pour into glasses.

# Healthy milkshakes

Another fine way to get extra fruit into small people. Straws compulsory. All these recipes work with soya milk too.

## Banana shake

Nothing but fruit, milk and a drizzle of honey. Just the way milk should be shaken.

Blend. Pour. Drink.

Serves 2
counts towards your 5-a-day

1 banana, peeled
250ml milk
a drizzle of honey
a pinch of ground cinnamon
   or vanilla seeds
3 ice cubes

## Chocolate milk with pear and ginger

The good people at Green & Black's sent us this recipe for our last book. We still eat as much of the stuff they make now as we did then. And we're still grateful for having this recipe in our lives today. Hence why we've included it in this book too.

In a small pan, gently heat the milk with the chocolate (broken into small pieces) until the chocolate has melted. Peel and core the pear and cut into quarters. Put the pear, chocolate milk and stem ginger into a blender and whizz until smooth. Serve warm or chilled.

Serves 1 generously
1 portion of your 5-a-day

200ml milk
40g Green & Black's 70%
   solids dark chocolate
1 ripe pear
½ a piece of crystallised stem
   ginger

## Orange and peach soya shake

This recipe uses soya milk instead of yoghurt. Perfect for those who are lactose intolerant. And for everyone else who likes peachy orangey soya-y drinks.

Squeeze the juice from the oranges and pour into a blender. Remove the stones from the peaches, chop the flesh into chunks and add to the blender. Add the soya milk and whizz until blended.

Serves 2
1½ portions of your 5-a-day

1½ oranges
3 peaches
150ml soya milk

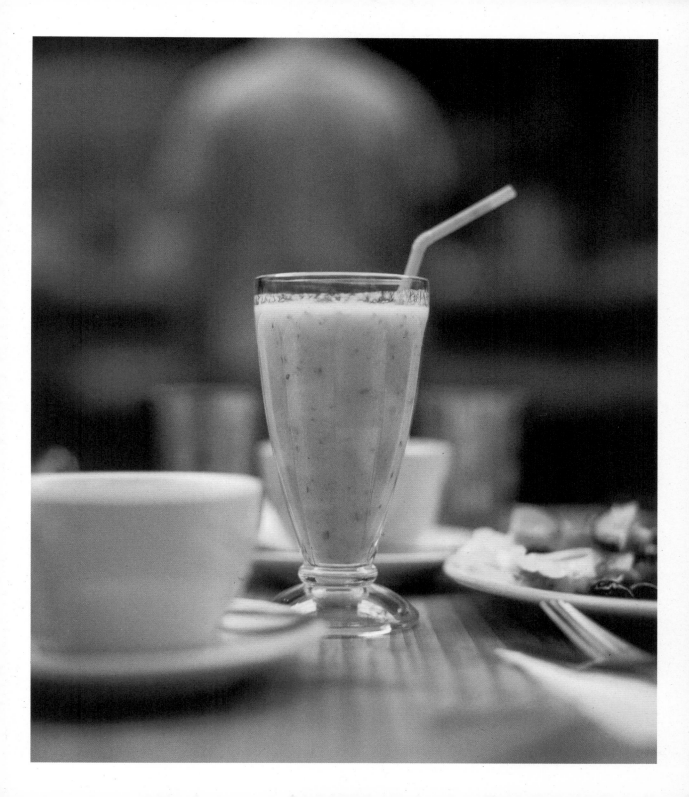

# Junior booze

Serve these drinks in champagne glasses or decant into one of those crystal decanters for proper posh pouring. I say.

## Raspberryade

Serves 3
1 punnet of raspberries
500ml sparkling water
1 wedge of lemon
sugar or honey to taste

There's bad fizzy pop and there's good fizzy pop. The bad stuff contains colouring, preservatives, sweeteners and other rubbish that kids don't need. The good stuff can be made at home from natural ingredients – see below.

Wash the raspberries and blitz them in a blender. Add the sparkling water and a squeeze of lemon juice and stir gently. Pass the mixture through a sieve to get rid of any seeds. Stir in a little sugar or honey to taste.

## Blackberry collins

Serves 2
1 punnet of blackberries
2 tablespoons of elderflower cordial
500ml sparkling water

A non-alcoholic version of the cocktail classic (first name Tom).

Blend the blackberries with the elderflower cordial. Spoon into champagne flutes, top with sparkling water and maybe add a little paper brolly.

## Peachy fizz

Serves 2
2 ripe peaches
1 teaspoon honey
500ml sparkling water

Like a Bellini but minus the booze. Muddle in a big glass or small bowl.

Remove the stone from the peaches and muddle in a glass with the honey. Spoon into champagne flutes and top with sparkling water.

## Elderflower cordial

Makes 3 litres
60 elderflower heads
2kg caster sugar
2 lemons

When you go a-elderflower picking, make sure you pick the berries that are looking at the sun. The amount of cordial you make depends on how many berries you can get your hands on. If you can pick enough, it'll see you through to next summer. Just make sure you have some clean glass bottles to store it in.

Gently shake the elderflowers to get rid of anything that might be hiding in there. Put the spiders back in the garden.

Pour 3 litres of boiling water into a really big pan, add the sugar and bring to the boil. Simmer for a couple of minutes, until all the sugar has dissolved, and take off the heat.

Cut the lemons into quarters and put them into a large bowl or a clean bucket with the elderflowers. Pour over the warm syrup, cover with a clean tea-towel and leave to steep for 24 hours.

The next day, strain the cordial through a sieve lined with muslin or a brand-new J-cloth into a jug. Pour into sterilised bottles, screw the lids on tight and store in a cool place.

To serve, mix 1 part cordial to 7 parts still or sparkling water.

# THE 10 COMMANDMENTS OF WASHING UP

## 1. Thou Shalt Always Use Hot Water

*Never lukewarm. Never cold. Boil a kettle if needs be.*
*Otherwise you'll just have to do it all again. You wash tepid, you wash twice.*

## 2. THOU SHALT ALWAYS CLEAN WITH GREEN

*Meadow fresh, pomegranate dawn, tropical sunset on the Costa del Sol. Best to stick with the green stuff*
*from the old school bottles. They still make the best rockets. Stay true, wash original.*

## 3. Thou Shalt Always Soak

*Burnt a pan? Lasagne stuck to the pyrex again? Douse in washing up liquid, cover with hot water*
*and leave to soak. Do this immediately or woe betide an evening of futile scrubbing…*

## 4. THOU SHALT START NEAT

*Pile the dirty crocks to one side. Insert plug or place washing up bowl in your sink, hold washing up liquid*
*bottle above and squeeze firmly for 3 seconds. Turn on hot tap, fill to bubbly and let washing up commence.*

# 5. THOU SHALT RESPECT THE ORDER

*Glasses first, cutlery next, then plates, chopping boards and less dirty pans followed by the stubborn bits.*

# 6 THOU SHALT NOT BLAME THY TOOLS

*Scourers for pans, scrubbers for other stuff, long-handled brushes for glasses, cloths for wiping down surfaces. Washing up gloves if you've just had your nails done.*

# 7. THOU SHALT HAVE FAITH IN THE METHOD

*Give everything a good wash, pile to one side then go back and rinse it all. Or rinse in sections to avoid the ire of your dryer upper. You'll save water, won't max out the hot tap or ever again suffer from soapy ramekins.*

# 8. THOU SHALT RINSE

*In case you were thinking of ignoring commandment #7, you must must rinse. Otherwise you're just pushing cornflake crumbs round a soapy plate. And life is too short to be entertaining soggy cereal.*

# 9. THOU SHALT CHERISH THY DRYER UPPER

*For they are the true heroes. Ensure you have 2 tea towels to hand, more if you're having a posh dinner party. And make sure they're clean. Not the one you wipe the cat's feet with.*

# 10. THOU SHALT SOMETIMES LEAVE IT TILL MORNING

*Because life is short.*

# thanks

thanks for the recipes

This is the third recipe book we've written but the first with anything other than just drinks in it. We couldn't have done it without the amazing Anna Jones. So biggest thanks are reserved for the First Lady of the Kitchen.

Then there are our guest recipe inventors – Lucy and Claire at Crumbs, Bronte at the Scandinavian Kitchen, Green & Blacks, Lizzie at Baby Organix, Ceri's mum Sian and, of course, innocent drinker Nadine Akle. Thanks for letting us use your excellent recipes.

Massive thanks also go to Sandrine Delabriere, Emily Ezekiel, Emma, the Mumsnet mums, Alison, Lucie, Ewa and her grandchildren, the lovely Carl and all the innocent folk who tested the recipes. Thank you for all being so thorough.

thanks for the photos

Clare took the beautiful photos with the help of Kitty, Tansy and Tyrone's spare camera.

Other thanks go to Chris Terry, the Greenwoods (Molly, Colin, Jesse, Asa and Henry) for letting us use their house, Tara, Ruby and Violet for giving up their Sunday, Rich, Melinda, Sally, Jenny and Pete for their respective kitchens, Sian, Steve and Jack for the Worcester retreat and all the cabbies who provided wheels.

Our models included our friends Hannah, Gus, Hildy, Freya, Luke, Hugh, Emily, Asa, Ruby, Tansy's pea boat and a rather haughty moose.

thanks for all the other stuff

Thanks to the innocent family for all their suggestions, Emilie and her dad for the translation, Aldworth James & Bond for the wood chopping, Kevin Smith, Scott Mosier, Adam and Joe and a variety of 80s hip hop kings for the backing tracks, Madhu for the juggling, Katharine for the yellow car and help and Meera for the jelly mould.

thanks for the guidance

Louise, Julian, Michelle, Sam, Rachel and the editorial tag team, Liz, Ione and Georgia, without whom there wouldn't be a book.

thank you

The biggest thanks goes to everyone who buys the stuff we make. Without you, we wouldn't be here. So thank you. If you want to stay in touch, join the family at www.innocentdrinks.co.uk/family. If you fancy working here, try www.innocentdrinks.co.uk/careers. And if you ever fancy a chat, come say hello at Fruit Towers, 342 Ladbroke Grove, London, W10 5BU.

# even more thanks

The pages in this book which are not recipes became known as 'The Distractions'. They were designed and written by some very fine folk indeed and we'd like to thank them for their time, generosity and talent in crafting such beautiful spreads. So to everyone below, thanks for making this book look hot. You're all ace and we salute you.

Things to do in 5, 10, 15, 20, 30 and 60 minutes (pages 34, 74, 156, 168, 212 and 308) Designed and illustrated by Marcus Walters, Ned Selby and Gareth White of New Future Graphic www.newfuturegraphic.co.uk Words by Ceri Tallett and Ben Williams

Have a butcher's (page 160) Designed and illustrated by Shaun Bowen of B&B studio www.bandb-studio.co.uk with the help of the proper butchers down at John Charles, 12 Blackheath Village, London, SE3 9LE

The remarkable tale of Ned the Newt (page 126) Words by Luke Bishop Design by Ben Williams www.bishopandwilliams.com

5 reasons to eat in season (page 114) Designed by Shaun Bowen of B&B studio with seasonal advice from Liz Cook www.thevegancook.co.uk

It's a conundrum (page 140) Conceived and designed by Harry Pearce from his excellent book 'Conundrums' (HarperCollins 2009)

Harrison and the prawns (page 276) Words by Ben Harris www.cargocollective.com/benharris Illustrations by Jim Smith www.waldopancake.com

Paints and potatoes (page 196) Designed and lovingly printed by Preston's finest – Claire Vickers Words by Ceri Tallett

The 10 commandments of washing up (page 334) and Eat your greens (page 206) Letterpressed and designed by Stephen Kenny at www.atwopipeproblem.com Words by Ceri Tallett

Tips from a Master Baker (page 280) Words by Andrew Whitley www.breadmatters.com

Doh Boy (page 285) Thanks to Pete and Ade at howies for letting us use Doh Boy www.howies.co.uk

The spotter's guide to pasta and things that go well with pasta (page 82) Illustrations by David Sparshott www.davidsparshott.com Words by Ceri Tallett

Robot food (page 219) Illustration by Rob Lowe www.supermundane.com Words by Ben Williams

Sunday night is alright (page 54) Photography by Steve Williams www.cygneturephotography.com Words by Dan Germain

Pie symbology 101 (page 136) Words and pictures by Ben Williams

Catch and release (page 144) Words by Tansy Drake and illustrations by Ben Williams

A guide to nicking stuff and leaving notes (page 290) Words by Molly and Rob www.weallneedwords.com Designed and illustrated by Kat Linger

# Index